Praise for the Author

Thank you Bruno for bringing me back what I really feel being the optimum me after many, many years of battling hormonal and weight issues, I am very grateful to have met you. You are very authentic and your diagnosis is very results driven. **Jey T.**

Bruno has a brilliant mind, I am just beginning to hear mainstream medicine speak of what Bruno was telling me 15 years ago. His supplements make a huge difference to my life. My arthritis has reduced significantly. **Margaret C.**

This is no fairy-tale. Following Bruno and Henriette's natural healing program my weight and life have already changed immediately. For all of you thinking about going down this path, don't waste any more time. DO IT. I promise you will not regret it. **Vikki H.**

I haven't felt as good as this about my life in a very long time. Now I have the energy and most importantly the motivation to continue with what I call a lifestyle change. I have told many people about you Bruno and will continue to do so. **Nicole A.**

With seeing Bruno my health has improved immensely. Now I feel amazing. People tell me I look amazing. I can't remember the last time I went to a doctor. When anyone tells me about their health issues, I tell them: "go and see Bruno". **Carla O.**

Bruno has always been supportive and with his exhaustive knowledge, I knew I was in good hands. The weight came off, my energy improved and my health remained excellent with the assistance of Bruno's carefully researched vitamin products and his excellent advice. **Roslyn B.**

Within two weeks of treatment from Bruno, The Marevich Way, I felt better than I had for 20 years. My energy levels are now like a teenager's, I'm much more optimistic and when I wake up I practically bounce out of bed, my energy levels are perfect all day, I'm regular and I actually look fresh and younger. I have spoken about Bruno to all my family and friends and know that some are also now getting help from him. I've got my life back. I really can't recommend you highly enough Bruno. **Leo L.**

After making an appointment with Bruno, changing my diet and taking some vitamins rather than antibiotics, my health has had a complete turnaround. I would never have imagined that I could feel so well within myself. It's one of the best things I have ever done. Life is too short to feel sick every day, I recommend your service to everyone. **Elizabeth C.**

My health improved quickly and has been stable for years. I have now been seeing Bruno for 10 years and would recommend anyone not having luck with conventional medicine to see him too. **Andrew B.**

Bruno was very understanding and explained in detail exactly what he would like me to do to achieve the results I wanted, The Marevich Way. Bruno is my saviour and I look forward to meeting with him every month because there's always something new I'm learning off him to help me along. **Antoinette A.**

I would definitely recommend Bruno Marevich to anyone who is willing and interested. I find Bruno's attitude to wellness and longevity motivating and inspirational. Also Bruno's availability to listen and explain clearly what is happening to me is much appreciated. **Gail P.**

Fifteen years later I still live my Bruno's creed, The Marevich Way, and understand our immune system is designed to heal us therefore a healthy attitude and following a healthy gut has kept my illness at bay and I feel 100%. **Glenn H.**

People often tell me that I look so well and ask me where I get my energy from. I believe Bruno's natural therapy has done wonders for my health and will still continue seeing him. **Pauline W.**

I've been seeing Bruno for 25 years on a regular basis. I believe I owe my good health over this time to Bruno. Whenever I have a health concern the first thing I do is go and see Bruno. He's never misdiagnosed my condition. **Pam McB.**

In about four weeks I had lost eight kilos by walking 40 minutes each day and following Bruno's diet and taking his supplements. I had not felt that good since I was in my teens. He has an abundance of knowledge and I am always confident in the advice he gives me. **Gary A.**

It's now been over 12 months since I first saw Bruno. Now I can't imagine not following The Marevich Way – his thoughtful advice and powerful supplements have literally changed my life for the better and we've referred a number of our friends to him. **Glen P.**

Bruno's wealth of knowledge and experience has been fantastic in providing a program that improved my lifestyle and made the symptoms either disappear or reduce to a manageable state. Bruno has a holistic approach to his treatment and provides clear explanations with his findings and treatments. We keep recommending Bruno to many friends and family. **Shawn A.**

Bruno diagnosed and treated my health condition by changing my diet and prescribed the right supplements, I am now back to working 14 hours a day, seven days a week. All I can say is "THANKS" and I would recommend anyone who is not well and has been unable to solve their problems to see Bruno and start enjoying the rest of your life. **Roland J.**

I would like to thank Bruno for his exceptional treatment and care in the last year and a half. After having had breast cancer and radiation I can say I don't feel as tired and I am a lot more energetic. I am looking forward to continuing treatment and future overall health. **Cecilia D.**

Bruno has always been there to support me through various on-going health concerns, both in person and over the phone. He has always offered a great deal of care, support and encouragement for which I feel so blessed. **Name provided.**

I have always tried to follow a healthy diet and lifestyle. However, in my mid-eighties I was diagnosed by a doctor with rheumatoid arthritis and prescribed dangerous drugs which I refused to take. I was fortunate to know the best naturopath in the world, my son Bruno. I am now 92, weigh a perfect 50 kilos and thanks to my son's directions and supplements I now live a fit and healthy life. Thank you son. **Diana Marevich**

Make Your
Health
GREAT
Again

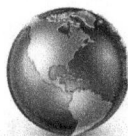

GLOBAL
PUBLISHING
G R O U P

Global Publishing Group
Australia • New Zealand • Singapore • America • London

Make Your Health GREAT Again

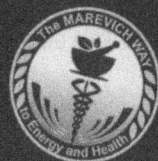

Find out How to Achieve Epic Wellbeing and a More Vibrant, Longer Life

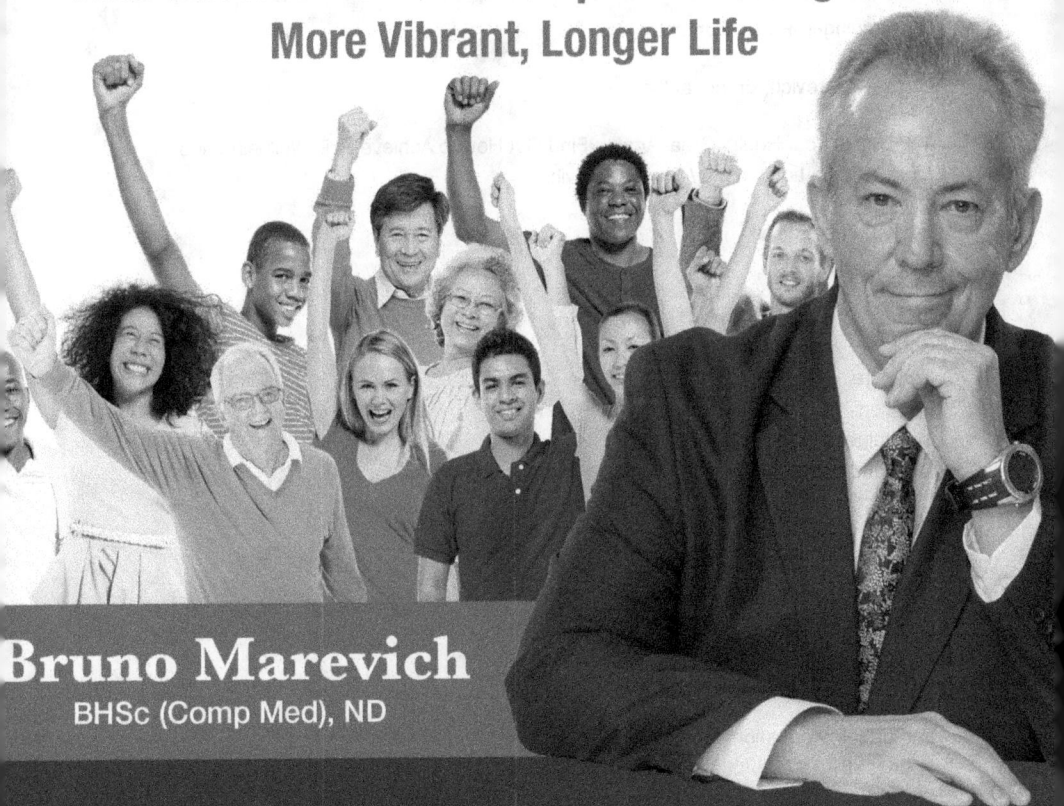

Bruno Marevich

BHSc (Comp Med), ND

Revealing The Marevich Way to Higher Energy and Superior Health, Naturally

First Edition 2017

Copyright © 2017 Bruno Marevich

National Library of Australia

Cataloguing-in-Publication entry:

Creator: Marevich, Bruno, author.

Title: Make Your Health Great Again : Find Out How to Achieve Epic Wellbeing and a More Vibrant, Longer Life / Bruno Marevich.

Edition: First Edition.

ISBN: 9781925288520 (paperback)

Subjects: Well-being
Self-care, Health.
Nutrition.
Mindfulness (Psychology)
Mind and body.
Conduct of life.

Published by Global Publishing Group
PO Box 517 Mt Evelyn, Victoria 3796 Australia
Email info@GlobalPublishingGroup.com.au

For further information about orders:
Phone: +61 3 9739 4686 or Fax +61 3 8648 6871

I dedicate this book to You, the reader, a very special being, conceived and made in the Creator's own image. You are a unique, essential and active part of this amazingly spectacular, eternal universe.

To all who are enjoying full good health, not so good health, at home, in hospitals, to those who are happy and those whose lives feel challenged at this moment.

To all who have sincerely committed their lives and continued efforts in helping others experience greater physical wellness and mental and conscious growth.

To humanity, every person of any age, race, creed, gender, nationality or social status. You have all been endowed with the seeds of greatness within you.

May all your lives prosper and become abundantly filled with great energy and health.

Bruno Marevich

Acknowledgements

I am very happy that I have been so fortunate in my life to have been able to get to do what I wanted to be able to do as far back as I can remember, since I was a little child. I felt then that my life's mission and desires would be fulfilled if only I could work hard enough at acquiring enough knowledge and expertise, so that one day this could help anyone who needed some of this knowledge and expertise, and they would want to use it to try and make their lives better.

I would not have been able to have helped so many people in my life unless I too had been so positively supported by my family and some other great people whose paths crossed with mine.

The first person without whom I would not be where I am and who I am is my dear wife, Henriette. She believed in me since the first day we met almost 40 years ago and has never ceased to do so. She is the source of my inspiration and motivation. She encouraged me every step of the way, at times even when I could have stopped and turned around. Our aims and drive are the same and she felt that by helping me unselfishly every step of the way, we could achieve our goal of benefiting the lives of others together. In the early years of our marriage she worked hard at casual jobs below her talents and abilities whilst also raising our children just so to make it possible for me to pursue my studies and profession. We have worked together at helping our patients since day one, are doing so today more happily that ever and look forward to continuing with doing so, even better if we can, for many, many years still.

My children, who have grown up listening to mum and dad talking about health and disease at the dinner table. It must have had some kind of an effect as Daniel is now a very dedicated operating theatre nurse and Ann a fabulous, caring dentist. We are proud that they are both doing what they love doing.

My mum and dad who always supported me and adopted a healthy eating lifestyle since we were children. Dad, a staunchly individualistic and very intelligent man, passed away a few years ago at the age of 91 and until not long before his decline had been exceptionally healthy with the best blood test readings of anyone I had ever seen. Mum is now 92 years young, lives with us, has no health complaints, is fully active, is as bright as a young lady, enjoys going for long walks lasting several hours with Henriette and I on a regular weekly basis and attracts the compliments of everyone she meets because of her youthful appearance and demeanour. She has long been a great living example of The Marevich Way which she does her best to follow every day.

Robert Lucy, a great Sydney naturopath and chiropractor who must have somehow sensed my desire to help people and have seen enough good potential in me to choose me, out of many, to take over his busy Sydney Macquarie Street practice and all his patients before passing away. He mentored me through my studies and early years as a naturopath. I always looked up to him and wished that one day I could be as good at diagnosing, treating and understanding people as he was. Robert passed away many years ago but I still remember all he ever told me. I have used his holistic philosophy of healing as the foundation onto which I added my own personal experience to create The Marevich Way which I continue to use daily with my patients in my practice.

Dr William Vayda, who has also long since passed away, whose traditional style of natural medicine philosophy closely interlinked to a strong scientific and medical basis. He made me appreciate the synergy of combining traditional with orthodox medicine which I strongly support to this day. He too believed in my potential.

I can honestly and gratefully say that I have stood on the shoulders of giants.

And this section could not be finished without acknowledging the countless number of patients who have given me the opportunity of doing what I have always wanted to do, help people live a healthy, happy, long and productive life, where they feel empowered to also help others and thus in a small but unstoppable way all contributing to the betterment of humanity.

Disclaimer

The intention of this book is to inform the reader of the author's observations, research and hands-on clinical treatments and experience over many years as a naturopath, as well as those of other scientists and health practitioners, which have allowed him to help many patients achieve better health.

Its purpose is to increase the reader's general awareness in the philosophy and practice of natural health treatment approaches backed by scientific interpretations and explanations where possible.

The scientific and naturopathic formulas, treatments used and diets contained in this book are only provided to give the reader general information and knowledge about the subject, and in no way to provide a complete, in depth explanation which would of course require more space than available.

Some of the comments and recommendations in this book may also be based on anecdotal evidence and not have been officially proven to full scientific and medical satisfaction as yet and thus may not be supported or recommended by medicine.

As every person is different, so is potentially the status of their health and the causes for their conditions, even though, when reading, they may appear to be similar to those of other people mentioned in this book. What may very well be correct for many may not only be unsuitable and indeed may also be dangerous for some others.

This book is therefore not intended to assess nor diagnose the readers' nor anyone else's state of health nor recommend any treatments, medications nor dietary requirements for which you should seek advice directly from a qualified, professional health practitioner.

My Gift to You

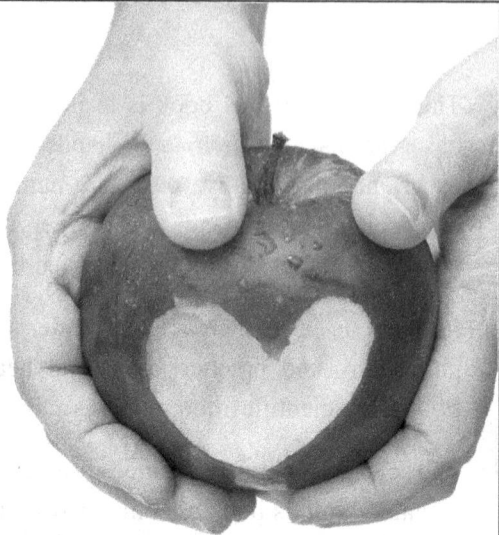

This book, *Make Your Health Great Again*, contains valuable information which has helped tens of thousands of people over the past three decades get over their tiredness, ill health and restore good energy and wellbeing.

To help you make it even easier for you to achieve this, we have made available for our readers a copy of our hypoglycaemic eating program, **The Marevich Way.**

Claim your FREE Bonus Gift by going to

www.TheMarevichWay.com.au

Contents

Foreword

It is a great pleasure for me to write a foreword for *Make Your Health Great Again: The Marevich Way to Energy and Health.*

I have been influenced by natural therapies from an early age through the influence of my mother who is a yoga teacher and a type 2 diabetic.

My brother and I grew up on a cocktail of fish oil and vitamins.

During my time in medical school as well as training and working as a GP in two busy practices I was able to see the tremendous benefits as well as limitations of modern medicine.

When it comes to chronic disease and autoimmune disease in particular the use of diet and lifestyle from my anecdotal evidence as a GP is huge.

We already know that type 2 diabetes studies have shown the benefits of diet and lifestyle on glycaemic control.

I have seen many success stories but also failures in terms of natural therapies during my time in practice. I think it is up to each patient to look at these therapies for themselves and search for the right practitioner to see if they may benefit from them.

The effects of supplementing with micronutrients, probiotics, lifestyle and diet on the gastrointestinal system and the immune system can be profound, even if difficult to explain.

As a doctor and a patient myself, I have seen firsthand the success of natural therapies used alone as well as in tandem with modern medical practice.

As with most things in life a middle ground is usually the safest and keeping an open mind always helps.

What may work for one patient may not work for another as we are all similar but very different genetic machines.

The present day lack of evidence based trials on such therapies makes it difficult for doctors as yet to endorse such practices however we are all on a journey and many patients will give natural therapies a chance having done their own research.

It is good to see a new book based on the long personal clinical experience and recommendations of an experienced naturopath, Bruno Marevich, give the reader even more well explained information and anecdotal case studies to provide more needed understanding as well as food for thought in the field of natural therapies.

The patient's good health always comes first.

Dr. Sanjeevan Nagulendran
FRACGP

Introduction

Are you and your loved ones fully enjoying those wonderful life's benefits that only good energy, health and wellbeing can bring?

According to the World Health Organization, good health is "Not merely the absence of disease and infirmity but a state of Optimal Wellbeing".

Too many people in the world today are sadly burdened with either medical conditions or undiagnosed health problems which often render them incapable to adequately enjoy all that life has to offer. Many others are fortunate not to be affected by illness or pain but lack the bounce and energy to fully embrace everyday opportunities.

'Optimal Wellbeing' can energise and fire our bodies, minds, hearts, deepest desires and beliefs and propel us to reach out, chase our dreams and bring them to fruition.

Medicinal drugs are sometimes important however they seldom fix the real causes of the condition and often only mask the causing problem. Untreated problems can and often do worsen with time.

The Cochrane Collaboration, the world's foremost body in assessing medical evidence, stated recently that "many of our most commonly used medical drugs are dangerous and are killing us off in large numbers". Whilst there are no clear numbers in Australia, in the United States an estimated 100,000 people die each year from the side-effect of "correctly prescribed drugs". Death from medical mistakes has now become the third highest cause of death in the United States following cardiovascular disease and cancer.

They have also found that although regular medical check-ups at your doctor may increase the rate of detection of cardiovascular disease and cancers, our biggest killers, it does not reduce our risk of dying from these conditions.

Prevention is therefore an extremely important factor, as many will agree that it is preferable to fix the pothole than having to repair the damaged car suspensions.

Most of us also agree about the importance of a good diet containing all the important nutrients essential for a healthy, vigorous and long life. Even the media often brings this to our attention these days; that health has become a popular and thus lucrative market.

"Eat all your vegetables!", you will often hear. Unfortunately modern intensive farming techniques, modifications to nature's balance and long hard-coded genetic wisdom, added chemicals, processing and refining techniques have all depleted vary large quantities of these essential nutrients from our groceries.

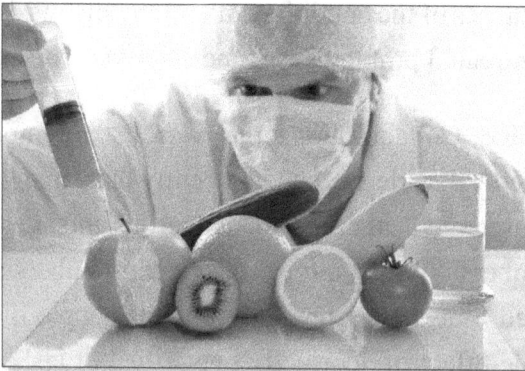

Today's fruits, vegetables, grains, eggs, even the milk and meats we eat are not even close to what they were a few generations ago. As an example, an apple a day 'used' to keep the doctor away. In 80 years apples have lost: 48% of calcium, 84% of phosphorous, 96% of iron and 82% of magnesium, the important heart nutrient.

> An apple used to contain almost half of our minimum daily requirements of iron. Today you could have to eat up to 26 apples each day to get that same amount.

These are shocking statistics as we are left with food, much of which is sometimes only useful to generate excessive oxidative stress for our cells and DNA, deplete our body's minerals and vitamins, destabilise our metabolism, disrupt our endocrine system, decrease our immune competency, make us more prone to all kinds of modern age diseases and deprive us of the optimal wellbeing essential to help us navigate successfully through life's experiences.

What's one to do?

The purpose of this book is to disclose and make available to everyone, a highly effective, health-restoring and peak-wellness promoting method, developed and used in our clinics over the past three decades.

Referred to as the 'The Marevich Way to Energy and Health' this method has been successfully prescribed, monitored and fine-tuned, in-clinic, with tens of thousands of satisfied patients. It has been used to help people with practically every type of sickness and condition whether well medically defined or 'mysterious'.

Time has come for us to reveal to you and the world this proven and intuitively logical natural treatment process for optimising and harmonising your body's major organs and systems.

Its purpose is to stimulate the spontaneous natural repair of the often unseen and unsuspected causative problems of most conditions or of suboptimal health. It endeavours to achieve this by putting your body back into a 'healing mode' rather than just helping with only the easing of the symptoms, to restore and optimise the function and performance of all our organs, our biochemistry and physical systems and processes. It takes advantage of our bodies innate, obvious but often overlooked ability to heal itself particularly when encouraged with foods which do not overtax its endeavours, natural vitamins and other forms of healthy medicinal quality nutrients and a healing mental attitude.

We wish to bestow upon the readers as much of our knowledge and experience in this field as is possible in a book this size, and to empower them with the expectations of greater energy, health and longevity.

> It has been our experience that in most cases
> the results from this type of treatment are often even
> greater than what the patients had hoped for.

Such are the advantages when treating the person as a whole and not just the presenting symptoms. It helps provide outstanding body and mind results not commonly experienced by most people and not usually achievable by other more common forms of alternative treatment or orthodox medical approaches alone.

Most of our patients achieve remarkable results and optimal wellbeing.

Also, by letting your professional health practitioner know that you prefer this form of treatment in conjunction with or instead of other more symptoms-oriented treatments, you are doing yourself and the rest of the world a favour.

CHAPTER 1

Never Too Late to Start Getting Healthier

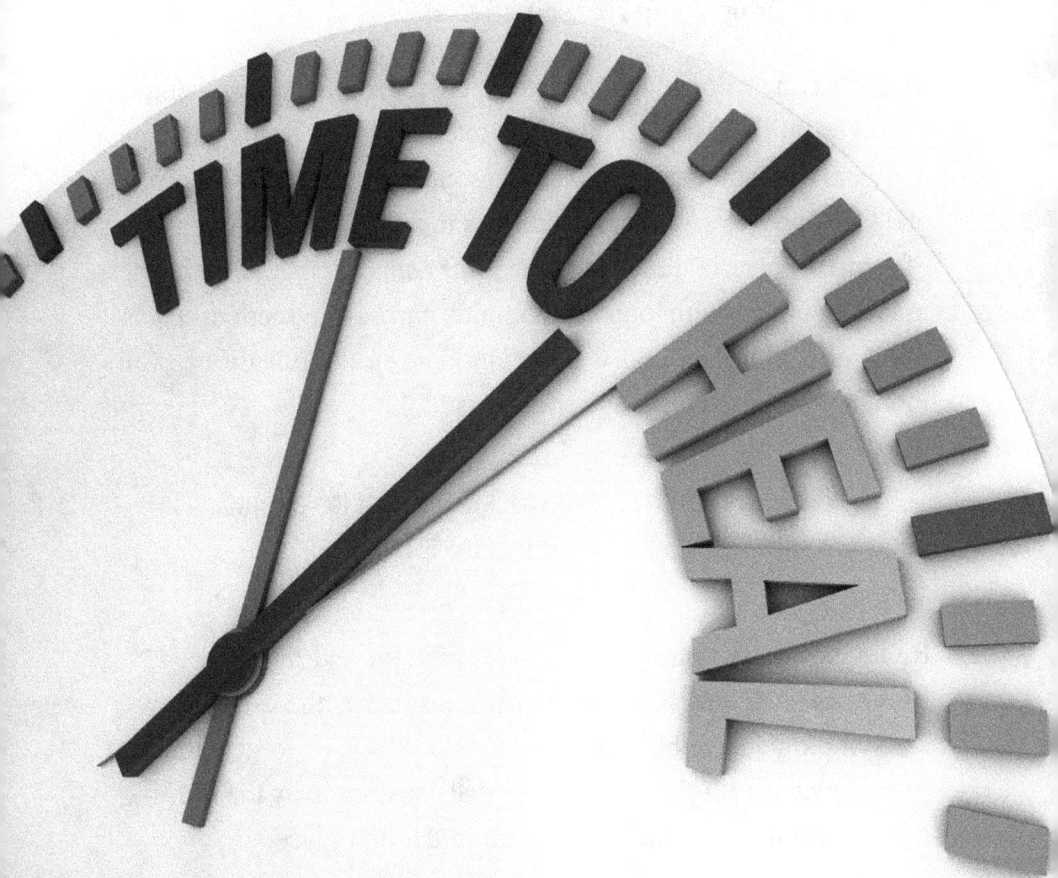

CHAPTER 1

Never Too Late to Start Getting Healthier

With several thousand registered prescription and over the counter medicinal drugs available from chemist's shops these days, we would be very justified in assuming that we are being attacked by an incredibly large army of diseases, all requiring very specialised 'antidotes' for us to survive their effects.

This is a conclusion that would not seem to be too far from being a real possibility if we even just tried to count in our heads the large numbers of manufactured toxins present in the air that we breathe and the water we drink. Also additives in our foods, different types of viruses, bacteria, fungi and other outbreaks of epidemic causing microorganisms with long and complex names that seem to spawn every now and then and which culminate in the release of even more new drugs and new vaccinations.

> I have always said, "Treat the causes, not just the symptoms". Never said "Don't treat the symptoms".

Relieving the symptoms is always important and may indeed be lifesaving. It seems however that in most cases these days, once the symptoms have been relieved, one neglects or forgets to also carry through with checking for the real causes of why the warning light was shining on their dashboard in the first place.

There are many times when during an emergency situation or a painful condition, the relieving of symptoms is absolutely essential. If you are having, say, a bad case of pneumonia, it will not help you a lot right now to sit around reflecting on the warning signs that your poor immune system may have been giving you for many years, or for regretting not having paid sufficient attention at the time by choosing to live a healthier lifestyle and perhaps having had lesser takeaways. Right now you should be immensely grateful to the hospital or doctor who have stuck a needle into your veins and is pumping you with antibiotics. This could very well have saved your life. However, it makes sense that the story would have been a lot better if you had taken greater care of your health in the first place. You would have had a much greater chance of the pneumonia not occurring in the first instance. However, because this can no longer be helped, what is done is done, you should decide to start taking better care of yourself once you are out of hospital and the emergency is over.

The same example could be of course used with practically every other health condition. If one has an advanced form of cancer, there may even be some advantage having the usual medical treatments which could include mixture of surgeries, radiotherapy or chemotherapy. One can't undo what has brought them here and at this stage, keeping alive is the most important priority and surgically removing a cancerous growth that interferes with the function of other important organs may at this point have become essential.

> According to the World Health Organization, up to 70% of some types of cancers can be blamed directly to poor lifestyle and nutrition.

In my opinion the percentage is a lot greater but let's go with official figures for the moment.

Also, the American Cancer Society says that "Nutrition is an important part of cancer treatment. Eating the right kinds of food during and after the treatment can help you feel better and stronger".

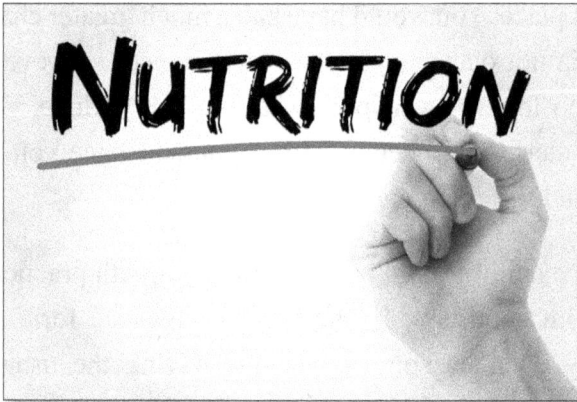

I would correct this statement to read "Nutrition is an *absolutely essential* part of your cancer treatment. Eating the right kinds of food during and after the treatment *may very well make the difference between winning or losing the fight* and *will* help you feel better and stronger". Also keep in mind that the right kinds of foods could have almost certainly helped prevent the cancer developing in the first place.

Do you think that this may be unproven or illogical and that only aggressive medical treatment will now help? Not so, according to many scientists and physicians. The statistics looking at survival rates after conventional medical treatment for cancer are disappointingly poor. It may prolong your life but just slightly and the quality of life associated with the treatment often makes one wonder if they would have been better off not having had the aggressive treatment in the first place. Most doctors have said that if they were diagnosed with terminal cancer, they would not pursue aggressive medical treatment which may only give them a 5% chance of surviving more than five years after the chemotherapy.

So, it is never a waste of time to start taking good care of ourselves, preferably whilst we still have our good health and youth to support us, or, during an illness to help us get over it sooner whilst, also helping to fix a lot of the problems that caused the illness to occur in the first place.

If we cannot or do not get the opportunity of eating well and starting with the right supplements during the course of our illness, and our condition may require emergency medicinal drugs or surgery, then, when out of danger, start making the necessary changes to ensure your health heads in the right direction from then on.

Case Study no. 1 – David's personal testimonial.

Having been diagnosed with Stage 4 diffuse large B-cell non-Hodgkin's lymphoma, I needed help from all angles.

Bruno immediately made dietary and vitamin recommendations, which we stringently adhered to. Chemotherapy was also part of the treatment plan, as drastic measures were required.

Prior to the commencement of chemotherapy, I saw my GP. He was so amazed that I had already improved even before chemotherapy, due to Bruno's recommendations; he wanted to see Bruno as a patient himself. Nowadays he also refers some of his patients to Bruno. We always found Bruno to be very supportive and encouraging.

When the chemotherapy treatment was completed, I once again attended Bruno's clinic. The improvements were most surprising. As chemotherapy is usually very harsh and destructive to the gastrointestinal tract, we believe the combination of diet and vitamins not only maintained, but improved my gastrointestinal tract, which also contributed immensely to a quick recovery.

Although you can never be completely confident, I am happy to say that I have remained Lymphoma free for two and a half years.

My wife and I are very thankful for Bruno's support and treatment.

David T.

COMMENTS: I have known David and his wife as good friends for a long time. The discovery of the advanced lymphoma was quite a shock, which David and Carolyn had to quickly come to grips with and suddenly change their lives even more to try and combat this serious condition. They were helped immensely by their strong faith, determination, positive attitude and Carolyn's perfect preparation, dispensation and orchestration of The Marevich Way supplements and dietary program.

Having the support of a really good doctor who was prepared to incorporate David's decision to include our supplements and nutritional help as part of his treatment also helped immensely. Having health professionals, who, although with different personal views and preferences, are prepared to set these aside and collaborate for the ultimate benefit of the patient, apart from the obvious synergistic health benefits, also takes away what is the very unnecessary and unwanted stress, and helps the patient remain focussed on getting better.

Again, the importance of the right supplements to improve the digestive tract's inefficiencies, and thus a very large chunk of the immune system together with proper nutrition, will always help anyone with any immune deficiency or other problem. Since his recovery, David and Carolyn are continuing to be focused on the correct nutrition, supplements and enjoying what they regard as up-building and valuable in their lives.

Because prevention is better than cure and in most cases prevention may help us by us never having to get to use extreme medical therapies, choosing to do something about our condition before we end up in hospital is of course a wise decision.

One of the problems with embarking on an illness prevention lifestyle, when there aren't any medical signs to warn us that we may be going in the wrong direction, is that it requires much greater motivation. Modern medicine is generally more focused on fixing something now when it is obviously broken that to have alerted the patient before the breakage.

The reason for this, in part, is that the usual complaints that people present themselves with at a doctor's or our clinic may not be that bad or dangerous enough as yet. People who, for example, are just tired, may get told by their doctors not to work so hard, rest more – or are sometimes left with the thought that it is all just in their heads.

Case Study no. 2 – Ken's personal testimonial.

I cannot thank Bruno enough for his guidance, wisdom, and professionalism in helping me overcome my health issues and put me on the correct path to a healthier lifestyle.

In September 2016, I went to Las Vegas with my wife and friends for a holiday. When on the plane I felt uncomfortable as my weight had again increased and I just felt unhealthy. I had always struggled with my weight, and would diet to lose 10 to 15 kilos, and then as soon as I stopped dieting I would put on the weight again in no time, and would usually put on a bit more. Along with my weight I was also insulin resistant; suffered and medicated for high blood pressure, and been prescribed Nexium for heartburn and laryngospasms.

I found Bruno's details and on the day I returned from my holiday in September 2016, I rang his practice, made an appointment, and I have not looked back since.

The combination of diet, vitamins and supplements has been easy to follow and maintain, and is not affected by my heavy workload and social life. Bruno's guidance in the correct foods to eat, matched with insights through eye diagnosis, have been spot on in helping me achieve and maintain my health goals.

It has now been ten months since my first visit and I have lost 31.5 kilos. I no longer take Nexium and have halved my blood pressure medication. I have not had a cold, flu or any illness that has been going around at work or home. I am no longer insulin-resistant, and my levels are under a third of what they were ten months ago, and my blood tests have shown a marked change for the better.

Now at 51 I am far more active and feel far better than I have for the last ten years. The diet has been easy to follow and I do not crave food like I used to. I have bought a pushbike, which I now regularly ride and have a new dog, Boris that I walk daily. I hate to think where I would be now if I had not come to see Bruno last year.

I have appreciated his knowledge, patience in explaining everything, and his down to earth manner. I look forward to my monthly visit/consultation with Bruno and Henriette.

I have recommended several family members and friends who are also achieving marked improvement in their overall health and wellbeing, which is the least I can do for the help Bruno has given me to make the needed changes to my diet and overall health, to ensure that I have minimised the risk of major health issues. Thank you so much.

Ken N.

COMMENTS: Ken is a good example of an intelligent, very busy professional person juggling between his clients and family life. He had already been aware for a long time of the importance of keeping his weight and health under control, which he tried to do, but no longer so successfully. The cracks were beginning to show in his health but not enough to warrant any serious medical intervention, just antacids and blood pressure checks. Had he kept going in the same direction, diabetes would probably have been the next bus stop. Diabetes, blood pressure, extra weight and indigestion add up to what? Heart problems, cardiovascular disease. Fortunately Ken did not wait for that to happen. His taking on-board The Marevich Way has brought him overall great improvements. Everyone sees it in him, everyone tells him about it, and many who are inspired want to do what he is doing. I should add that Ken's wife Sue is also on the same program and is happy to be gradually getting her particular health issues under control. Prevention is better than cure!

Other people have deteriorated to the stage where their health condition now has a name. It has been identified, usually through a combination of either blood tests, imaging tests or pathological analysis, to be a medical condition, and the appropriate drugs can now be prescribed.

Other times the treatment of recognised medical conditions may require more than simply drugs, as in surgery and other specialised treatments or interventions.

In these cases where the problem is already there, many people may find varying degrees of relief and stability through the drugs, others will struggle to improve and others unfortunately will get even worse. All these people will also be at risk of the potential side effects that accompany practically all drugs. The justification for the risk of the potential nasty side effects on patients is usually that they will be at an even higher risk if they do nothing at all.

Case Study no. 3 – Archana's personal testimonial.

I had been diagnosed with rheumatoid arthritis after having my second child. I was seeing my local GP who referred me to a specialist. Over the months I was prescribed with a combination of methotrexate once a week, a drug also used to treat some forms of cancer, Panquil, plus other anti-inflammatories and painkillers such as Panadol Osteo. Little did I know I was taking dangerous drugs which were slowing down my immune system and risking many other serious side effects.

I then saw a news article on TV where one lady died whilst taking methotrexate incorrectly. I had decided then this wasn't for me, as whilst it was meant to help combat my disease my general health was suffering. I would wake up feeling ill everyday with no energy.

My dad recommended me to see Bruno Marevich as he had recently already experienced great results with him in only a few weeks. This was a life-changing moment and I haven't looked back since. Bruno's natural supplements have helped me achieve a better quality of lifestyle. I have more energy than ever and feel better now that my body is free of toxins and my joint inflammation has almost disappeared. With a combination of taking the right supplements and the right nutrition I know that I am now getting the best treatment without the dangerous side effects. My family and friends can see the difference this change has made for me. I would like to thank Bruno for all his assistance and support during this whole process. I couldn't have done this without him always willing to take time and listen to my everyday issues.

Archana P.

COMMENTS: Archana is a young mother busily handling work, family and, up to not long ago, the pain and discomfort that come with the autoimmune condition of rheumatoid arthritis, where her immune system, the good guys, had decided to not only wage war with the bugs and other nasty things which could hurt her body, but to also her good tissues – in this case her joints. This causes great levels of dangerous inflammation and swelling. The same autoimmune process that hurt her joints is also known to cause problems with the eyes, lungs, skin, hearth and blood vessels as well as other organs.

Therefore Archana fell in the category of someone with a well-recognised medical condition that also has an established medical treatment plan.

The medications that were prescribed to Archana were intended to reduce the painful inflammation by quieting down her immune system. They were, however, also causing her unpleasant results and afflicting this busy working mum with lack of energy, fatigue and obvious worries and stresses about the possibility that her health may develop even greater problems down the road because of these side effects.

She knew that there were too many risks by just continuing with what at times appears to be the easier way of just taking drugs, which mostly just relieve the symptoms. Archana is now drugs free, practically pain free, overall healthier and happier, has recently started a new job and feels much more capable of dealing with her daily life. Archana will soon be placed on a maintenance program which consists of continuing with the healthier eating habits she has developed and gotten used to over the past number of months and some natural supplements to help her keep healthy and active with her busy lifestyle.

Naturopathy endeavours to: support and practice the sound and eternal principles of natural healing, including:

- **The healing power of nature:** the body has the inherent ability to heal itself. This vitality can not only heal, but restore and maintain health.

- **Treating the whole person:** health and disease result from many factors including physical, emotional, spiritual, environmental, genetic and socioeconomic ones. Within the body, the different systems are connected, dynamically balanced. 'Disease' occurs when the body is out of harmony, out of balance.

- **'First Do No Harm':** respect the inherent ability of the body to heal itself by using therapies that are non-invasive, gentle and safe.

- **Identifying and treating the cause:** illness does not occur without a cause, and symptoms are not the cause of illness. If the root of a problem is not corrected and only symptoms are treated, a more serious condition may develop later on.

- **Prevention is the best cure:** health is a reflection of how we choose to live. We help patients recognise their choices and how these choices affect their good health.

- **Naturopaths as teachers:** one of our principal goals is to educate the patient and encourage self-responsibility for health by building together with the patient a healthcare program unique to their needs.

> As natural healing benefits the whole body, there is no person with any known condition whose health will not benefit in some way or another from seeing a qualified naturopath.

In practically every case, also seeing a good doctor for more specific, in-depth medical diagnostics – including laboratory tests results and monitoring your progress as well as, if required, more aggressive forms of treatment – will generally give you the best combination of synergistic modern and traditional treatments and you will be able to expect better results. For emergency situations you should always see your medical doctor or hospital first, as there is no doubt they are better equipped to deal with life or death accident or similar emergency situations as well as some acute conditions.

Whenever seeing a doctor first, you should always express your desire for non-aggressive, side effects free treatments wherever possible and ask whether in their opinion seeing a good naturopath may be of help in further assisting with your condition. Whenever seeing a naturopath first, you should always ask how you should explain what they just told you to your doctor, so that the combined treatments will bring you the intended greatest benefits.

For a long listing of the more common conditions that we and many other suitably qualified naturopaths treat, you can visit our website at www.TheMarevichWay.com.au, or find these listed later in this book.

The combination of this book's introduction and this chapter so far will, by now, have given you some insight into the idea that natural prevention is always better than having to cure a health problem. There is nothing terribly new or revealing in these words, as shown by the fast increase of natural products and vitamins in the market over the last three or four decades. The growth is demand driven, and the demand is high and shows no signs of slowing.

None of this has gone unnoticed by the drug manufacturing companies which would of course prefer that one purchased their products instead. In Australia, the regulation for the manufacture of natural vitamins is practically as strict as the manufacture of medicinal drugs. This offers Australian manufactured vitamins the obvious benefits that strict manufacturing quality assurance protocols offer. Sounds like a balanced and fair deal you may think, and that what is good enough for the manufacture of drugs should also be applied to vitamins.

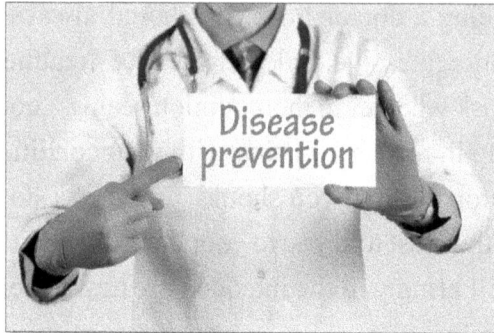

This may not look so balanced if you consider that hundreds of thousands of people die every year all over the world from the side effects of prescribed medicinal drugs. What does the official data show for deaths resulting from the use of vitamins?

> The American Association of Poisons Control (AAPCC) reported in 2011 that over the previous 27 years there had been 11 alleged deaths from either the side effects or misuses of natural supplements. A later analysis by the AAPCC revised this figure down to zero deaths.
> No deaths at all!

So the first question is whether it is necessary to apply the same levels of controls to a line of products that has induced zero fatalities over the last quarter century, as for one that has killed millions and millions of people over the same period of time.

One could answer that it does not hurt to be extra careful. And I would agree with that if the governments were also playing on an even field with subsidising your cost of buying vitamins as they do with drugs.

You can only buy cheap antibiotics, cholesterol drugs, blood pressure drugs etc., because like the pharmaceuticals benefits scheme (PBS) in Australia, many other governments in the world pay the larger portion of the cost of that drug from everyone's taxes for you.

So, could it perhaps be that the reason why vitamins are not more affordable and being pushed outside of the reach of all people including those in the less favourable socioeconomic backgrounds is the extra costs incurred in their manufacture because of not totally necessary controls?

Well, the present trend unfortunately isn't to relax the unnecessary controls and restrictions but to tighten them up, and it will probably continue to be so until you, the buyer demands access to better-priced vitamins.

Case Study no. 4 – Anna's personal testimonial.

My name is Anna and I want to thank Bruno for putting me on the right track to a better, healthier future. I am 52 years old and just over a year ago I started experiencing massive hair loss and extreme rosacea and acne (just to name a few things).

I visited my local GP (in the US) as I also have low thyroid, and thought that it may be the cause of my dilemma. My GP was very sceptical and tried to tell me that it was a combination of colouring my hair and reaching menopause. He nevertheless conducted the thyroid test I requested. A couple of days later he rang me and said "Congratulations, your tests are normal, you are perfectly healthy". I thanked him and then cried as yet another handful of hair came out when I washed it that

---

night. In desperation I spoke to a relative of mine in Australia that weekend and explained what had been happening. She advised that I go and see Bruno next time I visited, as he had done wonders in improving her health.

That was the longest five months of my life waiting to return to Australia so that I could see Bruno, as he was my last hope. In that short time, I had lost at least 50% of my hair and my face was a mess. Not to mention that I had lost my self-esteem and confidence.

Unlike your average GP, Bruno takes a holistic approach to healing the whole body, not just treating the symptoms. I have now been on Bruno's vitamins and diet for the last nine months and I am happy to say that I am sleeping longer without waking, my heart palpitations have stopped, some of my hair has started to grow back and my face has improved considerably. I also now try to take a healthier approach to the foods that I buy and eat, as I am more aware of the impact of healthier eating. I have kept in touch with Bruno by email and he is always very supportive and provides me advice and encouragement when needed.

If you know that your body is trying to tell you something, but your doctor says that you are fine, I would encourage you to try Bruno's method, which is safe and natural and a far cry from the treatments that the big pharmaceutical companies are trying to push.

Anna Mc.

COMMENTS: Anna's hair and skin problems would have almost certainly been contributed to by the hormonal changes which can at times have a strong effect on women in this age bracket, and also by her underactive thyroid which up to then appeared to have been kept under control with thyroid medication. Hair colouring preparations can also pose risks with the health of those using them. As another member of Anna's family was currently suffering with alopecia, one can only imagine the stress that thinking she too could be heading down that path may have caused.

The real problem highlighted in this study is that Anna's medical tests had all came up very positive and therefore, at least on paper, there were no obvious pathways at that stage to follow medically to seek a resolution for Anna's hair and skin, without perhaps having to results to other drugs. These may, perhaps, have kind of helped her hair and skin, but at what risk? And what about the real causes of her condition which were being left untreated? Same question about the underactive thyroid medication that Anna and many millions of people are on. They do not address the real cause of the problem which for the underactive (or overactive for that matter) thyroid is almost always caused by the immune system. The purpose of the medication for the underactive thyroid is just to give the patient a tablet which contains some of the thyroid hormones that the thyroid is producing in lesser quantities than it should. Works well in most cases, but what about the real culprit, the immune system that damaged the thyroid? What else can it do if it is not identified and dealt with?

Moral of the story: sometimes, as in Anna's case, medication may be helpful and may alleviate some of the bad symptoms which can make life so difficult. There is a danger however to assume that the problem has been fixed just because the symptoms have abated.

By treating Anna's underlying conditions her overall health has improved, her skin is much better and her hair problem has made a happy turnaround. The hair and skin made her look under the bonnet to try and fix the real problems.

CHAPTER 2

Pay Attention to Your Gut

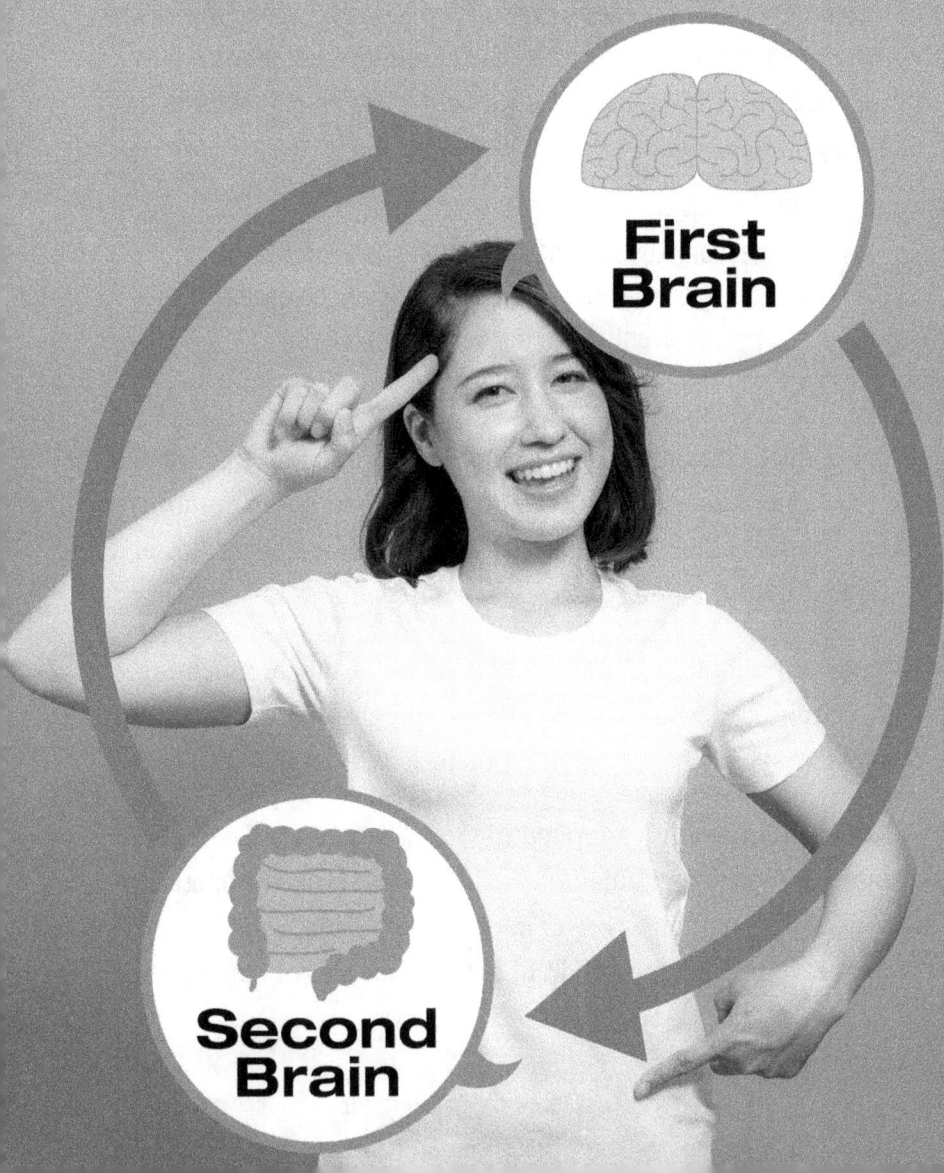

CHAPTER 2

Pay Attention to Your Gut

An exceptionally important cycle in our bodies to maintain health is that we must be able to digest our food, we must then be able to absorb into our blood the digested nutrients, vitamins and minerals, which must then be circulated by the blood throughout our bodies for cellular absorption, and then we need to be able to excrete – at cellular and intestinal level – what is toxic and no longer required.

> Digestion, Absorption, Circulation and Excretion.
> If there is a breakdown in this continuum, diseases
> will eventually manifest themselves.

There is little doubt that, of the whole body, the digestive tract is the most important and influential health promoting part, through which most people's present, past and future overall health and wellbeing has been and will be deeply affected.

Its poor or optimal function is responsible for much, much more than simply indigestion, wind and burping or reflux, the most commonly spoken of digestive problems.

A less than optimally calibrated digestive system will affect our immune system, our circulation, our heart muscle and its operation, and virtually every other organ in our bodies including our bones, hormones, brain and moods. In over three decades of naturopathic practice, I have never seen a patient in my clinic whose digestive tract could not be improved and who did not derive, sometimes to their surprise, measurable overall health benefits from my having done so.

The irony of it all is that most people are unaware of having any real digestive problems. They may normally agree that they may occasionally get some constipation, or diarrhoea or wind or some burping, "but everyone gets that".

Unfortunately the digestive tract is not always forthcoming with useful and accurate information as to its real condition and state of affairs. I have seen patients who thought that, sometimes with the help of the occasional antacid, their digestive tracts were working perfectly well, a conclusion sometimes derived from enjoying regular bowel movements or simply lesser reflux. And then one morning they noticed some blood in the toilet bowl, had it checked out by their doctor, had tests carried out, and all of a sudden are diagnosed with bowel cancer. The point is that most people are greatly unaware of what is going on in their digestive tracts, the very influential part that it plays in our good or poor health and our ability to recover from all forms of other diseases or conditions that may be presently affecting our physical bodies.

Fortunately, in the vast majority of cases, poor digestive tracts functions will of course not manifest themselves in the form of bowel cancers. They will, however, play a very prominent role in the starting and the supporting of a very large variety of diseases and health conditions.

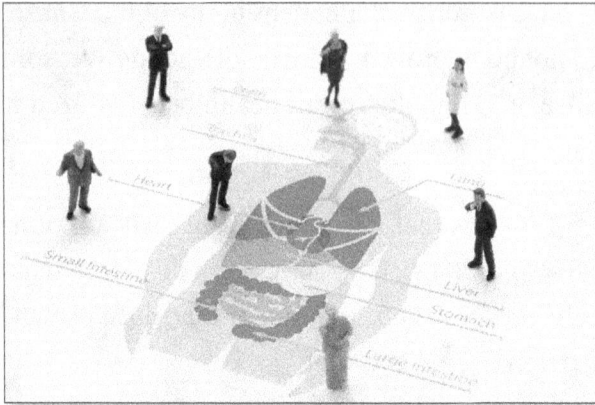

It makes therefore a lot of sense for every health practitioner to ensure, in order to obtain better results for their patients (and sometimes the only way to do so), that the taking care of the digestive organs and functions should always be a top priority. Sad to say this hardly ever happens in conventional medicine, nor as often as it should even in complementary medicine.

When was the last time that you or someone you know or have heard of, went to see their doctor because of skin problems or allergies or tiredness or insomnia or headaches or blood pressure or cholesterol problems or colds or irregular hormonal functions or virtually any other condition you can name, and got told by their doctor that they are going to help them by first working at improving their digestive tracts? Probably not very often. If a conventional doctor ever said that, you would probably look around and feel prompted to leave the room, wondering if you have walked in somewhere wrong by mistake. Or, you may not believe your ears and feel the urge to hug and thank them for the unexpected but intuitively logical advice and interest they have just demonstrated.

Case Study no. 5 – Rebecca's personal testimonial.

Since I can remember, I would feel quite bloated after eating certain foods. Over the years my symptoms worsened and I began to feel nauseous after most meals and would be in a lot of pain after eating. I was constantly going between being constipated or having diarrhoea. My anxiety sky-rocketed and began to control my life.

After giving birth to my third child at age 33, who was my third reflux baby, I initially sought Bruno's expertise to try and help my baby, as his reflux was causing him to choke at times. During my very first consultation, Bruno explained to me that my baby's reflux should improve if I fixed my own health issues, as my three month old son was surviving solely on my breastmilk at the time. Reluctantly, I took Bruno's information on board and walked away with my first lot of supplements and powders. I have never looked back since that day. I can honestly say that my life has been changed forever since that day.

I stuck to Bruno's diet and even though the initial first three weeks were extremely tough for a sleep-deprived mother of three to completely detox her body before the rebuilding could begin – the six kg I lost in those weeks helped me stick at it.

As the weeks went on, I felt like I had become a new person. I no longer felt bloated, I no longer had any pain and I didn't feel nauseous anymore after eating. I also had regular, normal bowel movements every day. Most importantly to me at the time though, was that my baby no longer choked! He was not only reflux free but he was sleeping longer, more soundly, and he was generally a much more settled and calm baby. What I didn't expect from following Bruno's diet and supplements was the rest of the benefits that would make me never want to return to the 'old me'.

Over the next few months I lost even more weight (nine kg all up) and I have never had more energy in my life! I don't feel the 3 pm slump anymore and my head has never felt so clear. My sleep has also improved greatly and I have been anxiety free since beginning Bruno's diet. Anxiety that I have struggled with daily for ten years prior to seeing Bruno. Gone!

My new found wellness has also had the most positive effect on my family. I no longer have mood swings and find myself to be a very calm mother and wife. I have not yelled at my children in months! I'm loving the newfound energy I have to chase after my three children, as well as the happiness I feel in general.

Who knew that treating my digestive tract's health could give me all of these positive effects? I certainly didn't. I cannot thank Bruno enough for giving me a whole new lease on life. I have no hesitation in recommending Bruno. He's been a lifesaver to me.

Rebecca S.

COMMENTS: Rebecca's eye diagnosis suggested low hydrochloric acid production in her stomach, damaged villi in her intestine and also hypoglycaemia or metabolic syndrome. By treating these causative factors, not only did her almost lifelong digestive problems practically disappear, today Rebecca feels happier, less anxious, even trimmer than she was already and more capable of enjoying her beautiful young family. From a medical standpoint her treatment may have generated the prescription of long courses of antibiotics and antacids to relive her tummy symptoms, which would have been unlikely to really fix the problem and perhaps hindered her digestive performance severely as well as antianxiety drugs. And what would have happened to the baby's reflux? Rebecca is following The Marevich Way and is happy not to have had to take any drugs.

So why, you may ask, are our digestive tracts so important?

Measuring some eight to ten metres – approximately five times your height – the digestive tract starts at our lips, travels through the insides of our bodies and terminates at the anus.

The digestive process often begins even before any food crosses our lips. Knowing that it is almost time for a meal, and thinking about and looking forward to consuming some delicious food, is often sufficient to get the digestive process started. Our brain, prompted by the alluring thoughts or sights or smells, assumes that there is a pretty good chance that we will be succeeding with obtaining some of what we are longing for, and proceeds to stimulate our salivary glands to start watering our mouths. Saliva, which contains a whole host of factors, not only water, and which softens the food for easier digestion later on down in the stomach, also contains its own form of a very important enzyme called amylase which is also found in a different form in the pancreas. Amylase helps digest some 30% of the simple sugars in our mouths before they even cross our throats.

The vagus nerve, which travels from our brain's medulla to our viscera, carries the messages instructing the stomach to begin releasing some hydrochloric acid. This is nature's own way of 'pre-warming the oven', so that some digestive enzymes in our saliva, as well as some hydrochloric acid in our stomach, are already on standby to begin the digestive process as soon as the food has entered our mouths.

The importance of reminding ourselves, our children or our patients that digestion begins in our mouth should never be considered underrated. Of course we all already know this, but honestly, given the pressures of time constrains and sometimes simply the instinctive habit of getting the food off our plates in a hurry, how many of us are consciously focused through most of our meal to eat slowly, chew well and only swallow when we have a mouthful of watery substance?

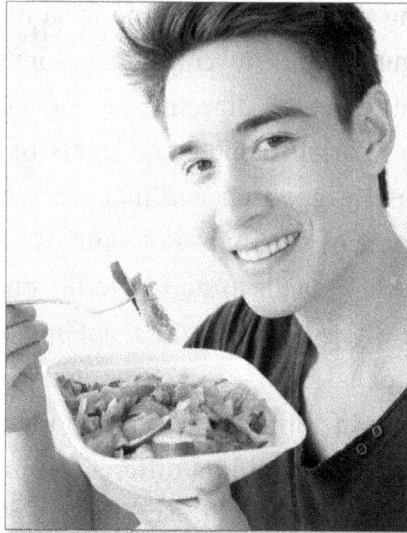

How often will we put the fork or spoon down after a mouthful and spend quality time pulverising and liquefying our food, whilst at the same time reflecting upon the content of what is in our mouths, tasting the flavours, enhancing the textures and linking these to good memories, happy feelings and a sense of gratefulness and appreciation? Probably not often enough.

And yet, isn't this what eating is meant to be about, and not just a process of feeding our intestines with the intention of being reminded by a full stomach that we are now ok, because we cannot stash away any more, and should thus stop eating until more space becomes available?

So, as our slowly and thoroughly chewed food, which has now been through maceration by our teeth and preliminary digestion by our salivary enzymes, gets swallowed, it travels down the oesophagus into the stomach, where the most important phase of our digestion is about to take place. This is also where a lot of confusion occurs, not only in our minds but also with modern medicine's evaluation and treatment of the problems that can arise from the stomach.

> Contrary to popular opinion which has taught us that the cause of many digestive problems such as reflux is because of the stomach's excessive acid production, with few exceptions, the truth is just the opposite!

Most digestive problems are actually present with people whose stomachs have produced hardly any good acid in years. Too little hydrochloric acid, also referred to as either hypochlorhydria or achlorhydria, is a condition officially recognised by medicine but normally, incorrectly, not perceived to be the real cause of most digestive problems for most of the patients walking into a doctor's clinic – other than perhaps those with cancer of the intestine. In reality, hypochlorhydria is almost always present whenever there is a negative imbalance between good and bad bacteria in the intestines.

Case Study no. 6 – Caleb's personal testimonial.

My previous history: Up until the age of 19 I had always been a relatively healthy teenager. It wasn't until I was struck with a severe case of gastroenteritis that I lost a significant amount of weight (approximately ten kg). Over the course of the next two years I remained unable to put any of the weight back on. This was concerning to me as my appetite was immense and I would often eat two to three servings at every meal, and yet never put any weight on at all. In addition to this, my immune system was virtually non-existent. I would get sick at least once every two or three months. I'm not talking about getting a little sniffle or a cough every once in a while. I'm talking about getting full on vomiting and diarrhoea, often complemented by a sore throat, headache and fevers.

This constant barrage of illness soon manifested itself into a form of chronic fatigue. I had started suffering at university and my grades were slipping. I knew something had to be done and so I started my quest to finally get to the bottom of why I was so ill all the time. I persisted with multiple visits to my GP, had numerous blood tests and was even referred to a gastroenterologist at one stage. None of these tests ever found anything conclusive. The doctors kept insisting that all of my results were 'normal' and that I was simply suffering from the 'flu' or some other virus that was going around. It wasn't until I was referred from a close friend to see Bruno that I finally got some positive results.

Bruno's treatment: (Month 1): I was sceptical about seeing a naturopath at first. Today's media often represents the practice as being far from evidence-based, often adopting a less than scientific approach to health and wellbeing. However, during my first consultation with Bruno all my doubts were cast aside. The initial consultation involved a brief medical/

health history and an explanation of the treatment approach that would be used. After hearing of my health history Bruno readily identified that my gut health was not up to scratch and decided to start me on his vitamins/medications.

He also, after performing a quick iridology review and pulse tracing/ECG, identified that I possessed a small heart murmur in one of my valves. The man had basically told me more about my health in a single one hour consultation than any of the other doctors I had consulted with for the past two years.

I'm not going to lie. The first few weeks of treatment were rough. I assume this was my body going through the 'detox' stage of my recovery. By the end of the month I had friends and family commenting that I looked thinner and more tanned in the face. I personally didn't feel or see any different to when I had first started Bruno's course, but I was determined to continue the treatment program to see if my health would finally improve.

(Month 2): During the second month I started to notice that my concentration was better throughout the day. I attributed this to both the vitamins/medications Bruno had given me as well as the strict diet Bruno had me following. In addition to this, my stools had now become so regular that I could predict when they would occur right down to the hour. During this time I also noticed I didn't get sick once (quite a remarkable improvement for someone as prone to illness as me).

(Month 3): By the end of the third month I FINALLY had my energy back. I would get anywhere between six and seven hours sleep a night and the moment that I woke up in the morning I would be full of energy, ready to take on the day. My concentration and energy soon translated over to my studies at university, which was quickly reflected in an improvement in

my grades. I also noticed that my skin had become slightly tanner (I no longer looked pale and anaemic) and I was in a much happier emotional state than when I had first started Bruno's program.

My health today: I continue to take Bruno's vitamins/medications to this day and am truly convinced of both their safety and efficacy. Thanks to his program I am now able to enjoy a happier, healthy life full of energy, focus, and most of all, a much more robust immune system! To say that Bruno has helped improve my health would be far from adequate. He is a life saver! My only regret is that I hadn't started his program sooner. It would have been far less expensive than all the medical costs I paid just to have doctors experiment on me with numerous diagnostic studies (none of which ever produced any helpful conclusion). Thank you Bruno!

COMMENTS: The fact that Caleb is completing his university studies to soon become a registered nurse may not be very surprising to the reader, given Caleb's well-accounted observations and conclusions. We are fortunate to see many nurses in our clinic who, like Caleb will soon be, are exposed every day to the suffering and other problems that illness generates and are thus gifted with empathy and a strong desire to see real healing take place, rather than only symptomatic relief.

Caleb's treatment with The Marevich Way focused primarily on repairing and regenerating his digestive tract and stabilising his glucose metabolism, and secondarily on supporting his immune system. As this started to happen, most of Caleb's other problems, headaches, fatigue, low immune system and all the problems that often go hand in hand with it, started to vanish and Caleb is now well on his way to enjoying ongoing good health.

Caleb's initial difficulty with detoxifying was to be expected giving his long history of poor health. Detox, or the getting rid of toxins, chemicals etc.,

etc. from our blood, intestines, liver and body's tissues can on occasion be a challenging affair, which at times requires our close supervision. That is why we make no exception of explaining to each and every one of our patients the reasons for detox and what they could experience, even though the vast majority will go through this process with only very minor inconveniences, if any, and start to feel the real benefits of the treatment very soon. It is generally the patients who react to the detox who will eventually be the happiest, meaning that there probably must have been a lot of stuff in the body that should not have been there and now that it has gone, they can feel the clear difference. We also provide all of our patients for the first month with free telephone support access and encourage/insist that they call if they have any questions, concerns or unusual reactions.

Higher than desirable levels of bad bacteria in the intestines are very, very common and I dare say that hardly anyone is totally immune from this problem in this day and age of refined foods, stress, and vast numbers of medicinal drugs, not limited to, but of course including, antibiotics. These medicines are sometimes very important, particularly in times of acute infections or emergency situations. They do however kill a lot of the good bacteria essential to good health as well as the infections causing bad bacteria, and the majority of doctors are becoming very aware of this. This leaves the intestines in a state known as dysbiosis where the natural biological terrain of the digestive tract has been thrown out of balance and there is not sufficient good bacteria left alive to limit the overgrowth of bad bacteria and other intestinal pathogens.

Imagine now the molecules in the food that you have just swallowed as a lump made of say many Lego pieces, held together by strong chemical bonds. These chemical bonds require breaking down so that the Lego pieces will separate and pass, separated, out of the stomach and into the first part of the intestinal tube, the duodenum.

The separation of these 'Lego pieces' from each other requires a good quantity and strength of hydrochloric acid. You may recall from your high school days that the strength of acids is measured on a pH scale where 7 is neutral (neither acidic nor alkaline). Pure water should have a pH of 7.

A pH higher than 7, i.e. 8, 9, 10 or higher is considered to be alkaline. Lower than 7 is referred to as acidic, with 0 being the strongest possible acid and being able to put dents and holes through metal. The pH of our blood is tightly regulated to be between 7.35 and 7.45, slightly alkaline. Even slight departures from this range can be very serious and life-threatening.

The hydrochloric acid in a good stomach should get down to a pH of between approximately 1 to 2, very low pH, and thus highly acidic, in order to successfully break the strong chemical bonds that hold the molecules in our food tightly glued together. Only then should the food in our stomach be released through the valve or sphincter at the exit of our stomach and into the duodenum.

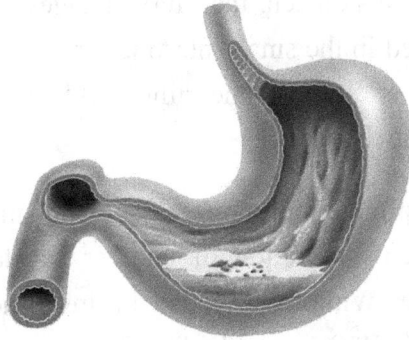

Sufficient amounts of high-strength hydrochloric acid (HCl) – which in my experience I have observed as desperately lacking in most of the thousands of patients both young and old who I have seen in my clinical career – play several vital roles:

- HCl is required to change a substance called pepsigen into pepsin which is required to help digest the protein in our food into smaller components called amino acids. A protein could be compared to a long train where each of its many carriages are a single amino acid. Each carriage must be detached or uncoupled from the rest of the train. That way, as an amino acid, it becomes capable of being absorbed through the villi in our small intestine into our bloodstream. The lesser the pepsin, the more is the absorption of the amino acids reduced. In general terms, there are at least 20 presently known amino acids and they are considered the building blocks of life. Almost half of these 20 are 'essential amino acids'. Essential, because the body cannot manufacture them from other substances and they must therefore first be present in our meals. The protein in our food is at first digested via our chewing, then by copious amounts of concentrated HCl produced by the stomach, then further digested by pepsin and finally absorbed in the small intestine through the villi into our bloodstream for delivery to the trillions of live cells that make up our bodies and who we are.

- HCl is in my opinion important by association in its participation of the stomach's secretion of another substance known as intrinsic factor. Without sufficient intrinsic factor, we cannot absorb vitamin B12 in our bodies. Lack of vitamin B12 can also lead to neurological problems, visual defects, weakness of the limbs, memory problems and even hallucinations and personality changes, as well as pernicious anaemia. Low levels of intrinsic factor are generally not considered by medicine to be caused directly with low HCl. In practice, I find that a stomach which is low in HCl is almost always, perhaps by association, also a poor producer of intrinsic factor. Many doctors regularly encourage some of their patients to have vitamin B12 injected directly into their blood. Many of these people will often report feeling better after receiving the injection. What neither party often realises is that the lack of B12 is very frequently due to, and a reflection of, the inadequate production of HCl in the stomach.

- HCl helps the absorption of iron in the intestine without which we can develop iron deficiency anaemias.

- HCl also acts as a barrier for unwelcome microorganisms which find it difficult to survive the passage through this acidic 'minefield'. The stomach itself is protected from the acid by a layer of mucus which is constantly secreted by the walls of the stomach.

- Low HCl can lead to many other nutritional deficiencies of not only amino acids but also other important nutrients such as magnesium, zinc, vitamin C, and B complex vitamins, which all participate in a wide variety of conditions, ranging from mild disturbances to life-threatening diseases.

Therefore, too weak or too little HCl acid will fail to achieve the adequate digestion of most foods which will cause partly undigested food to empty from the stomach into the duodenum.

If these food molecules, or the 'clumped Lego pieces' that have passed into the duodenum have been well digested and separated in the stomach to form a liquid slur referred to as chyme, they will be better able to undergo even further digestion whilst in the duodenum which will make them more easily absorbed by the millions of villi which line the intestine, into the bloodstream.

The further digestion of the chyme, whilst in the duodenum and before the final substance can be absorbed into the bloodstream, occurs firstly with the help of bicarbonates secreted by the pancreas directly into the duodenum. Bicarbonates are alkaline and help reduce the acid that the chyme has brought from the stomach.

The now less-acidic chyme can be further digested by digestive enzymes also secreted by the pancreas into the duodenum, as well as by bile secreted by the liver and stored in the he gallbladder, a bile reservoir pouch tucked underneath the liver. Good quality bile from the gallbladder and digestive enzymes from the pancreas thus complete the digestive process which allows the now fully digested chyme molecules to be absorbed by the villi into the bloodstream.

INTESTINAL VILLI

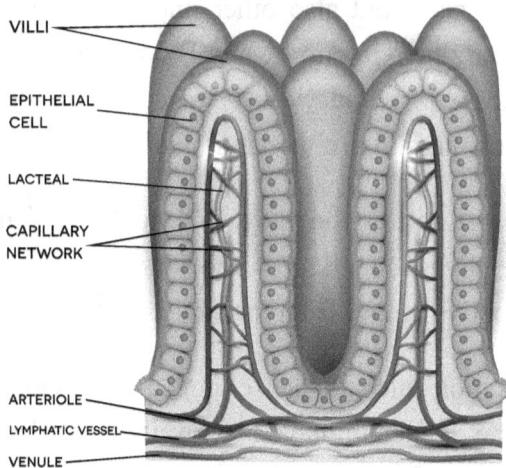

VILLI

EPITHELIAL CELL

LACTEAL

CAPILLARY NETWORK

ARTERIOLE

LYMPHATIC VESSEL

VENULE

Villi (plural) or villus (singular) are very clever little finger-like or hair-like protrusions that line up the small intestine. Think of them as hungry little straws that suck the nutrients through the walls of the intestine into the blood. The small intestine has several million approximately one millimetre long villi, and each villus carries thousands of absorbing microvilli. This vast array of villi and microvilli structures in our intestine dramatically increases the exposed area of the intestines available for absorption.

It is estimated that if all these folds in the digestive tract could be flattened and ironed out, our digestive tract could cover somewhere between an entire tennis court to a football field.

This is the level of importance that absorption plays in our bodies.

Inside of each villus there is a network of blood vessels which absorb the amino acids (digested proteins) and the glucose (digested sugars and carbohydrates) in the intestines, to channel these into our hepatic portal vein which then directs these nutrients to our liver for further processing before their end product is then transported to the cells of our body to satisfy their energy and nutrients requirements.

The inside of the villus also contains a network of lymphatic vessels which absorb the digested lipids (fats) from our intestines, and also transports them into our blood circulation.

The end result of low or inadequate HCl is that we may end up with poorly digested food regularly finding its way out of our stomach into the duodenum. If it cannot be absorbed, the food ferments, putrefies and encourages the overgrowth of bad bacteria and fungi. It is like throwing half-cooked food into the garbage bin – it will rot and attract flies, maggots and other disease causing organisms.

In the digestive tract, the bacterial and fungal overgrowth encouraged by the poorly digested and rotting food will create an unhealthy and toxic environment, and these undesirable organisms, the by-product of poorly digested and rotting foods, may then proceed with damaging the delicate villi structures.

Once damaged by the overgrowth of bad bacteria, the villi can become impaired and fail to carry out their filtering and absorption activities properly. This often results with the absorption of substances and organisms that would normally not cross the villi barrier into the bloodstream, a condition sometimes referred to as a 'leaky gut', as well as the poor absorption of vital nutrients which trillions of our cells require for their functioning and survival.

These substances often consist of molecules of ingested food matter which may not have been fully digested by the stomach into smaller components, or some of the overgrown bad microorganisms, toxins or antigens colonising and prospering in a now inhospitable small intestine, within which the growth of healthy, good bacteria has been hampered .

This leaky gut is a poorly recognised, but extremely common problem. It could be the cause of food allergies resulting in your arthritis, headaches, asthma, tiredness, inability to concentrate, multiple chemical sensitivities, irritable bowel and much, much more.

LEAKYGUT SYNDROME

The mucosal lining in the intestine, which separates the outside world from the inside world, is the most extensive and important mucosal protection barrier in our bodies.

When these not usually absorbed products have passed through this now damaged and leaking barrier of the intestinal lining and into the sterile blood, it now becomes the duty of our immune system to deal with it, and neutralise it if possible before this toxic matter can begin causing our bodies too much harm.

Case Study no. 7 – William's personal testimonial.

I wish to thank Bruno for the dramatic improvement in my health since I first came to see him. I am sure that there are many people who are in real trouble with their health and they are unaware of the existence of experts in naturopathy, or they are reluctant to try a new approach when conventional medicine fails to produce satisfactory results. I would encourage such people to do what I did and refuse to give up their search for good health.

Five years ago I suffered a stomach infection and I had to swallow 200 antibiotics in one month to kill the infection. Unfortunately, this killed off the good bacteria as well as the infection. I also developed high blood pressure and ended up on a very large dosage of blood pressure tablets.

The end result was that my stomach stopped working and this produced a very bad psychological effect. I could not sleep and my weight increased to 92 kg. I continuously consulted doctors and specialists to try to find a solution. I had one endoscopy and two colonoscopies but no solution was found.

Today, I have lost 12 kgs, I sleep well and I am on a very low dosage of blood pressure tablets i.e. 5 mg daily. I feel relaxed and healthy and, under Bruno's continuing care, I look forward to getting back to excellent health in the near future.

I had given up hope when I came to see Bruno initially. I was referred to him by a friend who was already a very grateful patient.

Again, thank you sincerely, Bruno. Without your expertise I am convinced that my health would have been in a terrible state by now. I welcomed the opportunity to do all the things that were necessary once I realised that you held the solution to my problems.

I would have no hesitation in encouraging people with health problems to consult with Bruno.

William M.

COMMENTS: William's case is a typical story where because of a really bad infection one has little option but to choose emergency medicinal drugs. Under the circumstances there was probably not a great deal of choice at that time when preventing the risk of greater harm with the infection being left untreated was the most important consideration.

Unfortunately, extensive use of antibiotics can have a dramatic unbalancing effect on our intestinal bacterial flora and in every other part of the body too. As well as killing off some of the targeted bad bacteria, the antibiotics will also bring extensive damage to the good bacteria which we require for our good health and a well-balanced immune system. Also, the more antibiotics we take the greater not only the damage but also the chances that we will be developing small pockets of bad bacteria which survive the antibiotics and eventually learn how to resist it. Antimicrobial resistance (AMR) is presently quite a worry in the scientific research and medical world, as the race is on to find new antibiotics before the current ones become practically ineffective.

The World Health Organization (WHO) released a report in 2014 stating: *"This serious threat is no longer a prediction for the future, it is happening right now in every region of the world and has the potential to affect anyone, of any age, in any country"*. Also, according to the Centers for Disease Control and Prevention, *"Each year in the United States, at least 2 million people become infected with bacteria that are resistant to antibiotics and at least 23,000 people die each year as a direct result of these infections."*

What we can learn from Williams's personal experience is therefore that taking care of our intestinal condition, including our intestinal flora and good bacteria should be a constant priority before infections or other type of health problems occur.

The advantage of doing so is that we will have a greater chance of avoiding infections that may routinely be treated with antibiotics, but also a greater chance of not needing too many antibiotics in case there is an infection. As most common infections are self-limiting and likely to get better by themselves anyway, if offered antibiotics, ask the doctor "do I really need them?"

CHAPTER 3

Your Gut Will Take Care of You

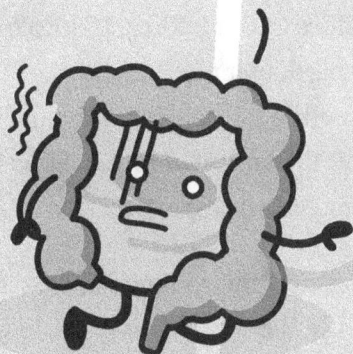

Unhealthy

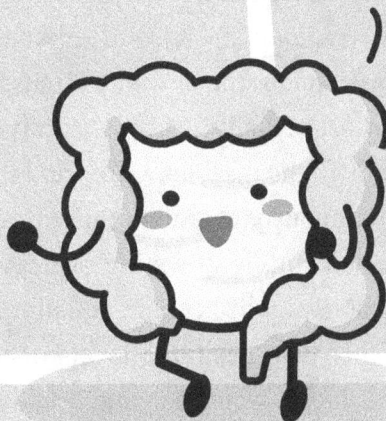

Healthy

FINISH

CHAPTER 3

Your Gut Will Take Care of You

> Most people don't realise that some 80% of our immune system – our body's friendly protection army – is found, of all places, in our gut

Quite rightly so, because this is an important 'customs point' between the outside world and the insides of our bodies. If 80% of the world's armies were stationed in a particular place in the world, one would be right to assume that something of major importance is taking place there and also that any unwarranted provocations could culminate in undesirable and dangerous responses.

So, as poorly digested food molecules and microorganisms pass into our blood through the damaged villi, the immune system, like a good defending army, does what it is intended to do and in various ways attacks the unwanted transgressors. Nothing wrong with any of this, actually it keeps us alive. However, if this transgression through the disabled villi – and the need for the immune system to continuously deal with this extra unintended work – becomes too demanding, long lasting or heavily focused, the immune system responses will become equally aggressive. This means releasing higher than desirable levels of immune substances in our blood and tissues which can and usually do become problematic, not just for the toxins but also for our unsuspecting body organs.

This provocation of the immune system causes a demand for extra soldiers and monitoring agents, spies, to be present at the border, due to the excessive arrival of unrecognised aliens through the broken gaps in the intestinal barrier.

The immune system then engages in the activity it was created for, to attack and kill these potentially dangerous aliens, for the purpose of defending us from any harm they could cause. Whilst in worldly confrontations of this magnitude there would probably be guns, bullets and bombs, the protagonists in this battle are a complicated array of immune responses which include the release of inflammatory agents such as histamine.

These exaggerated immune defensive activities, and the release of inflammatory agents, at first will more than likely make us susceptible to developing different levels of the more common types of allergies. Some people seem to become more prone or sensitive to sinus conditions, some to asthma, others to different types of respiratory and skin allergies.

Over the years we have successfully helped countless cases of skin problems, such as eczema, dermatitis, psoriasis, acne and rosacea without ever, ever, using any creams or other skin treatments. Many of the patients will have seen skin specialists, who will have often recommended anti-inflammatory drugs, perhaps gaining some immediate but usually not lasting results.

Whilst anti-inflammatory medicines will calm down some of the overreacting immune system activities and thus improve the symptoms of the respiratory or skin allergy, it will not cure what in my and many others opinion and experience is usually the true cause of the inflammation or the aggravation of the inflammation, the leakage through the intestinal wall.

> I normally refer to skin problems and other allergies as red lights shining on the instrument panel of a car. They are not the causative problem, they simply alert us that there is some kind of a problem under the car's bonnet

It is not sufficient to only cover or remove the warning lights on the dashboard, otherwise the purpose of the warning will probably go ignored while the real problem may remain untreated and risks eventually becoming more than a simple disturbance.

This inflammation manifests itself in the form of a variety of different conditions in many people, such as digestive complaints, joint and muscular pain, fatigue, difficulty with focusing, mood changes and the usual seasonal allergies.

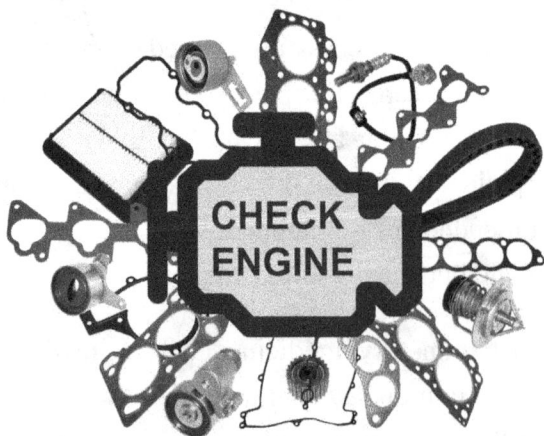

Other times, the sufferer of an overactive immune system may not be afflicted with or be aware of any particular allergies. However, there is always a very real risk that the overstimulated and belligerent immune system may actually make mistakes and confuse healthy tissue organs, such as for example the thyroid, with some kind of alien molecule which should not have, but did, pass the damaged walls of the intestinal barrier.

The immune system would now have learned how to attack this type of molecule or pathogen, which may have had some similar characteristics in common with the thyroid tissue and it now starts thinking that the thyroid is also an alien that's needs attacking. Gradually, the poor innocent attacked thyroid becomes damaged by antibodies from our immune system and begins either producing too much or too little of the important, metabolism-regulating hormones it is meant to secrete into the blood, sometimes leading to hypo- (Hashimoto's) or hyper- (Graves' disease) thyroidism, classed as autoimmune diseases.

There is a long list of some 80 or more autoimmune diseases that create a multitude of different problems and suffering, and in general terms they all have to do with an overaggressive or mistaken immune system attacking the otherwise healthy organs in our bodies which it was meant to protect – all more or less acting as in the above example used to describe the thyroid disease.

Autoimmune conditions are quickly becoming a scourge of the modern world and are estimated to affect a staggering 50 million Americans.

They include conditions such as reactive arthritis, rheumatoid arthritis, lupus, scleroderma, Sjogren's syndrome, vitiligo, several gut conditions such as celiac disease, ulcerative colitis and Crohn's disease, type 1 diabetes, multiple sclerosis, and the list goes on and on. The medical treatment for those autoimmune conditions often requires the prolonged use of nonsteroidal anti-inflammatory drugs (NSID's), corticosteroids, immunosuppressants and painkillers. Again, these drugs, like almost all others, are capable of serious side effects. They will generally alleviate the symptoms but in the longer run, at times, the side effects may be worse than the condition they were intended to treat.

Case Study no. 8 – Shelley's personal testimonial.

When I found Bruno Marevich I had very severe allergies and hay fever that were gradually getting worse and impacting heavily on the life of not only myself, but my family. I could even hardly do anything, or go anywhere outside, as I would be ill for the rest of the day/week.

Bruno's diagnosis of me was astoundingly accurate. He asked me to tell him in one sentence only what the main issue was that I was coming to him for. Then using iridology, he began to accurately list all the heath issues I had and even some past issues. He claimed that he could help me with these, and he was correct.

I began the detox treatment right away. This involved a combination of supplements and diet and lifestyle adjustments, The Marevich Way. The more dedicated you are to following the regime, the better the results. It is an adjustment at the start, but becomes a normal lifestyle as you go along. A couple of weeks after starting this treatment I found that I was not needing the array of hay fever and allergy medications that I had

---

been surviving on for years. Six months later I have almost forgotten about the pile of things I was previously taking to just 'survive'. Such a dramatic change!

There were many other benefits too I began losing weight, something I hadn't been able to do, no matter what I tried for years. In fact I was just continually putting on weight even when I tried to lose it. Six months later, I now have lost a total of 17 kg. Also, my immune system has kicked into action again. I no longer get every bug that is going around. My circulation has vastly improved. Bloating, a continuous upset tummy and diarrhoea has disappeared and my energy has returned. I feel like I have a new lease of life.

My husband was so impressed with the results I got that he began changing his eating habits and he has lost 5 kg now too. My daughter has been seeing Bruno as well with similar dramatic results. Thanks Bruno.

Shelley S.

COMMENTS: Shelley's rapid improvement from her allergies, her improved energy, younger and fitter appearance and healthy weight loss can be again attributed to the cascade of benefits that occur when the digestive tract and blood-sugar metabolism are assisted to work in the way they were intended to. Shelley's determination to get better after not having really felt on top of the world for some time, and sticking well to her treatment protocol, The Marevich Way, caused her to quickly see improvements after improvements. A great achievement and a very motivational case, as Shelley's improvements also motivated her daughter, who I also see as a patient, to improve her own health. These days they are both finding it normal to enjoy healthy foods and take a maintenance dosage of health sustaining and disease preventing natural supplements.

This is what can happen once our digestive and absorption dysfunctions have upset parts of this vital agent in our body, the immune system, our police force, bodyguard and army that has been made responsible for protecting us against nasty viruses, bugs, all kinds of toxins and damage. The companion with whom on our side we have walked confidently through places that contain diseases such as hospitals, and who has protected us since when we were little children playing happily and digging the dirt in the ground with our bare fingers. It is now doing something which we would never really expect a friend and protector, to whom we owe so much gratitude for looking after our best interests for most of our lives, to do.

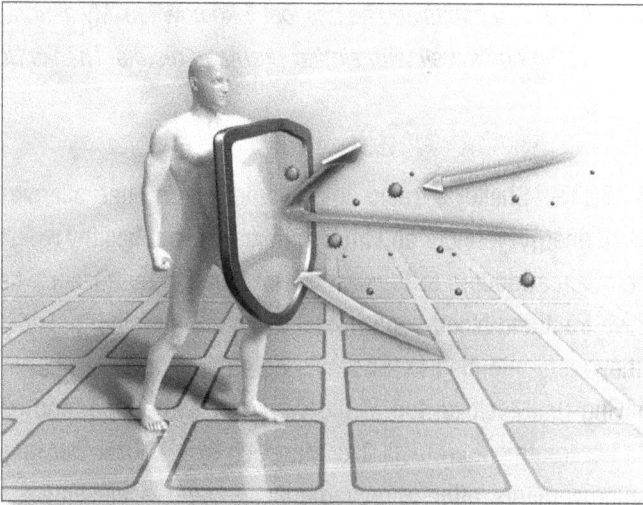

Well, the immune system should not really be blamed, as it is usually not the culprit but really the victim, whose great power for good has been damaged mainly by modern day foods, stress, environmental factors and the overuse of potent medicinal drugs.

But the problems do not end here because the damaged, leaking villi, do not only allow the passage of bad stuff into the blood – to add insult to injury they also block the passage of important nutrients which would normally get through without any problems, often causing subclinical, and thus often not easily detectable, malnutrition.

In my clinic I will usually no longer bother, unless I think it appropriate, to do all kinds of test to see if we can figure out exactly what the patient is not absorbing when I also suspect villi damage. Just supplementing the patient with the ingredient they aren't currently absorbing is no guarantee that the patient will be able to absorb enough or any of these anyway.

Very often, the damaged villi could fail to absorb many nutrients including B group vitamins, certain amino acids, essential fatty acids, iron, calcium, etc., etc., and there is no single organ in our bodies, including our very important heart and brain, that will not risk becoming seriously impaired.

We could walk through any hospital anywhere in the world and look at the medical history and profile of each and every patient in every ward, the cardiac ward, cancer ward, renal and dialysis wards even the psychiatric, neurology and emergency wards, and find out that with the exception of the maternity ward and some patients in the emergency ward, most beds would have never been occupied if that person or their health care provider had taken good care of their digestive tract along the lines explained in this book. Also, a large percentage of the remaining hospital patients could be safely dismissed if sent home and had these disease causing digestive factors worked on, as they would gradually be overcoming the real reason for their having become ill in the first place.

That is also why practically every person walking through a health practitioner's door will almost certainly be also burdened with digestive issues, sometimes for many years, and yet they will have rarely, if ever, been diagnosed or treated. These issues will almost certainly be the not-so-obvious, real, original causes of the seemingly unrelated health problems they have come to seek assistance for. If not, whatever the original cause of the condition, such as perhaps a virus or some other form of infection or injury, a well-functioning and unburdened digestive system will always promote better, more complete, faster healing and recovery for most patients.

For a multitude of reasons, most people either do not chew their food adequately, or their stomachs are not capable of producing good quality and quantity HCl, or have poor bile production due to sluggish livers, or lack in the essential nutrients which are required for their pancreas to produce copious amounts of health bringing digestive enzymes and bicarbonates – or perhaps even all of the above. Add a diet containing a multitude of refined foods with unhealthy and sometimes dangerous additives, and possessing little if any nutritional value, drinks, stresses, a vast variety of prescribed or over the counter medicinal drugs and, ouch, what a mess we have.

This may sound amazing and perhaps even hard to believe but it is very much so. Not only I, but countless other naturopaths and professional complementary health care practitioners, scientists and professors will have records of patients they have treated or researched and studied with such conditions. In our case, over the last three decades we have been fortunate to been able to assist restore good health in tens of thousands of people where normal medicines did not appear to have been able to, by prioritising the correct, health producing and maintaining function of the digestive tract.

The aim of every good health practitioner should always be to help their patients achieve a level of actual healing and not just relief, to minimise recovery time, reduce the patients need for drugs and give them, wherever possible, even greater health benefits, rather than just fixing the problems that brought them to their clinics. This should also be an opportune time to empower the patient whilst they are there, with valuable information to help them and their families prevent future similar or related health problems.

> Treat the causes, not just the symptoms.
> How much healthier would our world be if this
> were to happen?

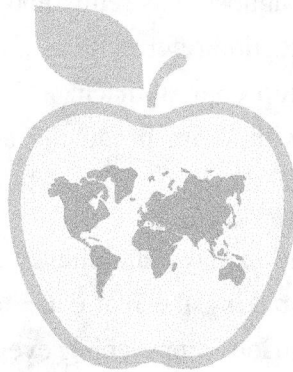

But the greatest irony of them all is that all of these bad bacteria in the intestine will more likely than not also produce certain amounts of bloating causing gasses. Some patients get so bad that they report getting bloated with almost anything that goes into their mouths, even water.

The pressure from this bloating can travel upwards as well as downwards. The upward travel finds a natural blockage, the valve or sphincter, that locks the acid inside the stomach. However, if we have overeaten – and sometimes also without eating but have perhaps done some lifting – the gas manages to escape through the weakened sphincter, pick up what little acid most people have in their stomachs, and splash it up past the stomach into the oesophagus.

This reflux condition will generally create some burning and discomfort but not always so. Some forms of reflux are silent and may only affect our throats, teeth or breathing. Others are not silent at all and can cause such sharp abdominal or chest discomfort that may easily at times be confused as a heart attack. Either way, your doctor will usually diagnose it as reflux and recommend that you take antacids or medication referred to as proton-pump-inhibitors which pretty much stop your stomach, which was not producing much acid to start with, from producing any more real usable amounts of required acid.

So, whilst the medication may help relieve the symptoms in many cases, it is actually making the real cause of the problem even worse. Now, the stomach is producing even lesser quantities of acid and is failing to digest food even more that it used to before, encouraging even greater overgrowth of bad bacteria, greater passage of unwanted molecules and toxins into the bloodstream, making it even more difficult to absorb the good essential nutrients and weakening and damaging our health even more.

Case Study no 9. – Zdenka's personal testimonial.

I started seeing Bruno after years of living with really bad bloating and it was starting to really affect my everyday life. I tried to eliminate foods from my diet that I thought were causing my bloating with no such luck. In the end I was so frustrated about my constant pregnant-looking belly that a friend suggested I go see Bruno, as she had seen him for similar symptoms.

So I finally made an appointment with Bruno and it was the best thing that I've done for my health. Thinking that I was fit and thinking I was eating mostly healthily, Bruno made me see that I wasn't eating the right foods, and that was why my bloating was never subsiding.

After suggesting I be on a balanced diet, plus taking the natural supplements, I started noticing a big change with my bloating, it was subsiding dramatically and to top it off I was losing weight (all in all I lost nearly ten kg) without trying!

Now after nearly three years I still see Bruno every few months. I've kept my bloating at bay, and have maintained my weight loss, and have implemented my healthy eating with my family at mealtimes.

Zdenka D.

COMMENTS: As in Zdenka's case, abdominal bloating is a sign that our gastrointestinal tract is filled with air or gas creating a feeling of fullness and tightness leading to swelling or distention of the abdomen and is sometimes accompanied with pain, flatulence, rumblings and burping or reflux. With Zdenka, some RRR (remove the bad bacteria, replace it with good bacteria and repair the lining of the intestines) brought rapid improvements to the symptoms, even though it took several months to achieve good repair and stability of her digestive tract. These disturbances can become so regularly bothersome as to eventually cause people's abdomens to become very easily distended after eating just about anything. Whilst bloating is normally reported as just an uncomfortable nuisance, it is really a warning that there is some degree of imbalance in progress in our intestines which could well be affecting our overall health, University studies have found that people suffering with bloating take more sick days, have to see their doctor more frequently and take more medications than the average person.

Bloating is something that you should not simply disregard, even if you consider it as just an annoyance. It could be a warning light trying to make you aware of certain food intolerances or sensitivities or even more serious conditions such as tumours, celiac disease, pancreatic insufficiency or even ovarian cancer.

Practically every patient that I have ever seen who was taking acid-inhibiting drugs has no longer required them, and been able to stop taking them in a few weeks and often much sooner and have never had to go back to taking them again.

How do I do that? It is often as easy as 123 or 'RRR'.

- **Remove,** using natural means that do not harm the good bacteria, the bad bacteria, fungi, yeast and mould from the digestive tract. There are many herbs and vitamins that will help do this. We find that using our formula, which contains the combination of a very potent dosage of active garlic extracts and horseradish combined with natural anti-inflammatories such as fenugreek, quercetin and bromelains, will get rid of most bad bacterial and fungal overgrowth, including help control the dreaded ulcer-forming helicobacter pylori.

- **Replace or replenish** the existing low counts of good bacterial organisms with appropriate amounts of health-giving good bacteria. Our preferred probiotic formula has high counts of colony forming units (CFUs) of the right strains of acidophilus, bifidobacterium longum, and higher than commonly available counts of bulgaricus, and also importantly contains prebiotics such as oligo fructose, which provides nourishment for the live encapsulated bacteria, and facilitates its prolonged survival, as well as their colonisation and growth in the small intestine.

- **Repair** the damaged villi, the mucosal lining and thus the immune capacity of the intestine. A combination of herbs will generally be able to help achieve this, such as slippery elm bark, aloe vera, fennel, ginger, liquorice, white willow bark, chlorella and guar gum, a mucopolysaccharide which in powder form helps coat and repair the cells and tissues lining the intestine.

While the total number of living cells that make up the living organs in our bodies is difficult to estimate, because of their differing sizes and concentrations in different organs, and many studies have proposed different numbers, it is probably not too wrong to estimate that there are a staggering 100 trillion living cells in our bodies, all with specific needs and functions and requiring proper nutrition and energy management.

Imagine you're being the owner of trillions and trillions of little factories, all responsible for different functions, each working independently, at full steam, each equipped with all the machinery and systems to enable them to perform their important job, and yet all synchronising and cooperating to achieve the grand goal of a healthy life.

If the figure of 100 trillion living cells sounds like a figure that we may not even be able to grasp in our minds, then consider that we also have an estimated quantity of intestinal microorganisms, which is some ten times higher!

The biological soil of our gut is comparable to that of a healthy, massive garden, beaming with life and activity. We are really the rulers of our own massive, purposeful universe and we are also born with an innate desire of being a good and wise ruler, which we further develop as we experience and learn from life. A good ruler has a deep interest over the running of his massive domain, and endeavours to protect it from questionable outside influences and enemies, and also seeks to learn how to make better informed, more valuable decisions that bring peace and prosperity to his subjects.

Therefore, as far as you can, keep this private universe well maintained with your best intentions for it, and expose it to the most beneficial and natural products that you think will be of benefit and not harm.

> Digestion, followed by Absorption, Circulation and Excretion. If there is a breakdown or inefficiency in this continuum, different diseases could eventually manifest anywhere in the body.

If your digestive tract is not healthy, neither is the rest of your body. If healing is at a standstill, look at the digestive tract to see if it is holding you back from getting healthier.

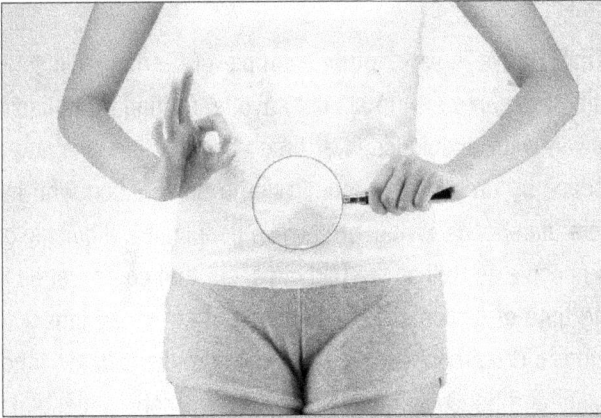

At least, in a simplified way, this is how our digestion and absorption process was intended to and should work for good energy, health and wellbeing.

Case Study no. 10 – Lyn's personal testimonial.

A few years back I spent more time in hospital than I did at home. I was suffering from an allergic reaction to an antibiotic prescribed to me. I was unable to travel far from home and working was becoming increasingly difficult.

The doctors prescribed stronger and stronger medication, all unsuccessful. I took to the internet and found Bruno's website and decided to give him a go.

The effects were almost immediate, I was back in control and I've never felt more alive. My colleagues at work are amazed when I don't come

---

down with colds and the flu. I can't thank Bruno enough for restoring my health and keeping me well.

Lyn M.

COMMENTS: Lyn is yet another example of the negative side effects that antibiotics can cause in almost anyone. Getting rid of bad bacteria aggressively with antibiotics is at times comparable to trying to bring world peace by dropping an atomic bomb on a nation who has more dissidents than peace-loving, productive people. It will quickly get rid of the good people as well as the bad ones, but that could just be the start of a long time of discords that could also affect many other countries. Continuing to drop more atomic bombs will make it harder and harder for stability and peace to be ever reached. In many patients, including Lyn, an unhappy intestine affects the immune system negatively, sometimes almost immediately, and this can lead to a vast variety of immune reactions, including respiratory, skin and intestinal distress. An immune system caught up in such a civil war will usually be far less able to protect the body from outside opportunistic invaders such as colds and the flu, or other allergies such as sinusitis or asthma. There is only a thin border between the outside and inside world. If that border gets broken, you can expect responses from your immune system.

CHAPTER 4

Love Your Liver

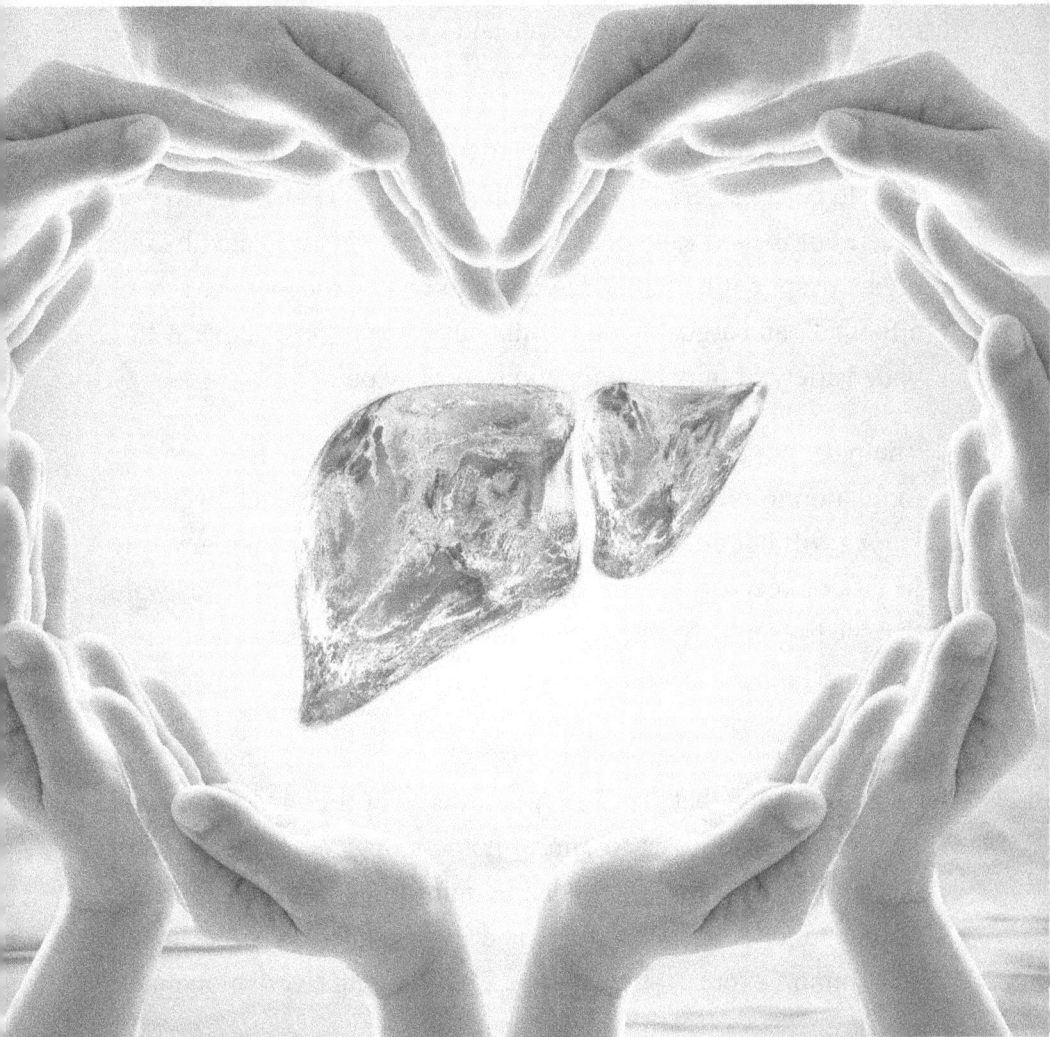

CHAPTER 4

Love Your Liver

The best advice that I could give you for a long and trouble free life is to 'love your liver'. If we look after our livers and take good care of them we will live longer and our life will have far more zest and joy.

Of all the topics to be discussed at a friends' gathering, the liver would have to be considered the lowest in popularity. Understandably so because it is hard to look at a liver and feel very attracted by this organ, despite it being the largest in the body, roughly the size of a football, and arguably one of the busiest and most active with a wide variety of important functions to carry out.

The most popular reference at parties regarding the liver may be in relation to the excessive alcohol consumption which everyone knows will not do our liver any favours. nor enhance in any way its task of keeping us healthy. Apart from that, some will be aware that the liver may be responsible for the not so brilliant cholesterol readings on their last blood test.

Deep down however, we all suspect, even if not knowing the exact functions that the liver performs, that a poor liver cannot be a good health asset to aim to possess, and we have all heard the concerning side effects that certain drugs have on the liver, of alcoholic livers, fatty livers and liver cancers. The no longer so common expression as it once was, 'feeling liverish' includes feeling disagreeable, nauseated and irritable. However, despite our liver often 'talking to us' to give us feedback on its condition, most people often will not suspect that their feeling ordinary is linked to their liver, until their blood test returns elevated readings on their liver enzymes.

The most common messages that a dysfunctional liver may send us will be in the form of constipation, flatulence, fluid retention, headaches, abdominal pain or swelling, itchy skin, dark urine colour, loss of appetite, chronic fatigue, pale or bloody and tar-coloured stools, and at its worse jaundice, cirrhosis or cancer.

> The liver is estimated to be performing a staggering number of over 500 functions.

These include the storing and metabolising of sugar in the form of glycogen together with fatty acids and proteins, as well as of the fat-soluble vitamins A, D, E and K, also vitamin B12, and the minerals iron and copper; filtering our blood; creating bile for digestion and storage in the gallbladder; metabolising important hormones; filtering as well as purifying and clearing of toxic waste products and drugs; synthesising proteins such as prothrombin and fibrinogen important for blood clotting and albumins which are essential for maintaining the right environment in our blood to ensure the right balance of water in our cells, as well as cholesterol and sugar.

The liver also plays an important role as part of our immune system through the Kupffer cells, a type of white blood cell only found in the liver, which assists us to maintain our health, by capturing and destroying bacteria, fungi, old blood cells and foreign substances that have found their way in the blood because of injury or illness, or simply worn out cells due to the normal ageing function.

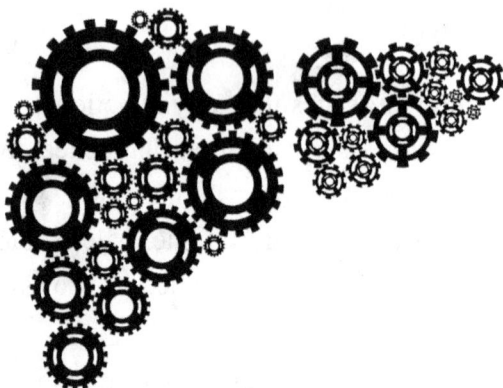

Despite being so busy carrying out so many tasks, the liver still remains capable of regenerating itself quite quickly, so in most cases of toxicity (including alcohol), by stopping taking it, the liver will often recover and the patient will feel well again. In fact the liver has the greatest capacity for regeneration than any other organ in the body. You could lose up to 75% of your liver tissue and the 25% remaining healthy liver cells will be able to regenerate the lost tissues again.

Our present lifestyle, nutrition and environmental factors seriously affect the liver by placing enormous stresses upon it. The pesticides which enter our food cycle, food colourings, plus an increasingly large number of chemicals that can be added to foods, means there are estimated to be as high as some 40,000 different substances that the liver may need to deal with. These have a gradually increasing detrimental effect on the liver the older we become.

Children's sensitive livers become affected too and it is natural for parents to be worried as their children fuss and pick their way slowly and with difficulty through healthy foods, such as protein-containing foods. When the liver is not healthy the person usually lacks appetite, feels full and prefers junk food, which does not contain any substances that have to get the liver too engaged, cereals for breakfast being one example, and nutrients lacking snacks during the day another.

Without healthy nutrients, a liver cannot produce bile of the correct pH. Without bile we cannot digest and therefore absorb and excrete our foods properly.

Many of my patients when asked at their first visit what they would normally eat for breakfast will often say either sugar-loaded cereals or perhaps not even that, but just a cup of coffee, usually using excuses like "I am too busy" or "I do not normally get hungry until after lunch time". Not surprisingly, when I tell them that their breakfasts should consist mainly of healthy animal protein, I will at times get strange looks and hear comments like "Protein? Are you sure? How ghastly!" This is unfortunately often just an indictment on their liver which is still deeply asleep in the morning and just the thought of consuming protein is enough of making them feel sick, let alone eating it. The concept that they can easily eat a large meal for dinner, often late in the afternoon or evening and then just go to sleep with it in their stomachs appears to make more sense than starting the day the right way by eating a healthy egg.

This poor eating pattern then induces further health problems, and so gradually one body-system after another begins to malfunction and eventually breakdown. Adults grow to rely more on cups of tea or coffee laced with added sugar to raise their own sugar levels and fire up their energy by borrowing on their adrenal glands. We are breeding a more and more 'liverish' population of poor or non-breakfast eaters, who are mostly tired, fatigued or exhausted and cannot focus until mid-morning, lunch, or after a cup of coffee.

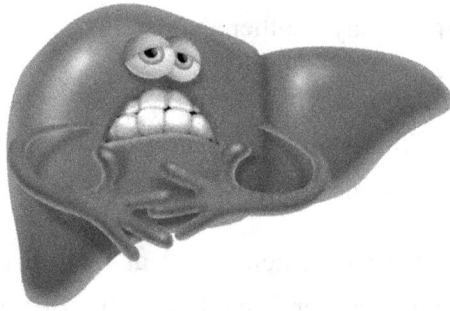

To maintain adequate liver function the nutrients methionine, choline and inositol are required in sufficient quantities. Their protective influence against damage to the liver is invaluable. Methionine can be used again and again in an enormous variety of nutritional reactions within the body. Without methionine and choline, cholesterol is not changed into bile acids and heavy deposits are laid down in the arteries, fats are not burnt for energy and lecithins are not produced for cell and nervous system utilisation. Without sufficient methionine in the bile acids, duodenal ulcers may form. It has been demonstrated that during infectious diseases the production of white body cells, lymph cells and antibodies has been substantially increased by the addition of methionine in the prescribed treatment.

If fingernails split, are thin, break off, won't grow or are spoon-shaped, the sulphur containing amino acids such as methionine may be needed.

Chronic constipation may occur unless sufficient bile salts are produced to keep the chyme emulsified on its long passage through the small intestine and large colon. As more and more moisture is extracted from this material the further it travels, it is essential to keep it well softened with bile of the correct pH. Otherwise hard lumps of insoluble soap are formed from undigested fats. Colitis and diverticulosis may appear and pain and inflammation is then present. Chronic cystitis and nephritis affect millions of women and indicates a condition of kidney damage, but the liver may be the real culprit.

The liver nutrients methionine, choline and inositol may help prevent this problem and correct long standing cases.

The lack of ability by the liver to metabolise fats because of insufficient methionine, choline and inositol means that Vitamin A is not utilised and dead epithelial cells may clog kidney tubules. Infections may then occur.

Puffiness and darkness under the eyes, headaches, frequent burning urination and high blood cholesterol may occur. These symptoms may be reversible by utilising the correct combination of nutrients. Help yourself to sensible living, eat plenty of vegetables, raw or lightly cooked, some fruit and animal proteins.

> Contrary to popular opinion, juicing is not as good for you as you may have been told.

Juicing predigests the fruit and vegetables thus liberating the sugars and even worse, fructose into the watery substance. Apart from lifting sugar levels quickly and making you more predisposed to adult onset diabetes, the liver will not get as much benefit from the juicing as you may imagine. The liver is a bowl of grease and requires sulphur containing amino acids which are found in animal protein such as fish, meats, poultry and eggs to energise the liver's cells, the hepatocytes to perform their functions well and perform their work efficiently.

Also, as known since ancient times and confirmed by hundreds of clinical studies, the herb silymarin, a flavonoid derived from the milk thistle plant, has been shown to possess hepatoprotective qualities, i.e. protect the liver against practically all types of damage, including damage induced by viral hepatitis, as well as hepatitis induced by toxic agents and radiation.

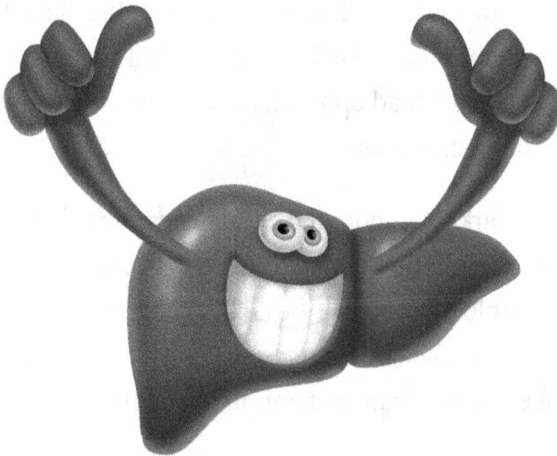

Its uses as a liver protectant, decongestant, carrier of bile, cleanser of liver and spleen and in the treatment of jaundice and gallstones can be traced back to the ancient Greeks and famous Middle Ages herbalists. It has been also proved to help both liver and kidney cells repair and regenerate.

Alcoholic and non-alcoholic fatty liver disease, insulin resistance and oxidative stress are major pathogenic risks, leading to the injury of liver cells. Long-term studies of the administration of silymarin showed significantly increased survival time in patients with alcohol-induced liver cirrhosis. It has also shown to protect the liver from chemotherapy-induced damage, making it less toxic and more effective for the liver as well as protecting it from metastatic cancer.

This herbal extract does all this with little risk for the patient.

Case Study no. 11 – Ingrid's personal testimonial.

In July 2013 a small tumour was discovered on my liver; as months passed the tumour grew in size, as did many changes to my body such as weight gain, constantly feeling tired and not being able to eat much food without being sick. February 2014 I had the tumour removed along with half my liver and gallbladder. The surgery was tough as it could not be done through keyhole due to the size. After ten days in hospital I was able to go home and back to normal life. Thankfully the tests showed it was not cancer. As the scar healed and the body healed the weight did not drop off, even though I was hardly eating anything as I was either sick before I ate or after a couple of mouthfuls. The doctor and the specialist said just give it time and my diet shouldn't change and I should be able to eat like before, as the surgery would not change my eating habits.

As month after month went by I noticed eating was harder and I didn't want to eat, as it was easier not to so I wouldn't be sick. But now other signs were staring to show that something wasn't right within me. Yet the doctors and specialists said nothing was wrong. I just couldn't shake the feeling that I wasn't healing as I should.

Bruno Marevich was recommended to me and I thought I had nothing to lose as I had tried everything else, and why not meet him and see if there was anything that he could do? I had never been to a naturopath and I thought it would be perfect as it could be more natural, as the doctors only wanted me to take tablets and medications.

I went to my appointment with an open mind and a list of concerns as long as my arm. I had concerns with my food and not being able to eat or being sick when I did, constantly feeling tired and fatigued, feeling light-headed and having no energy, depression started to affect me. I was up and down with emotions, my hair was falling out, my nails wouldn't grow and were thin and brittle. I constantly had a sweet taste in my mouth, my legs were constantly sore and muscles were sore, I still had a lot of pain also from the surgery as well as not sleeping well so I guess you could say I was feeling pretty sick all the time.

Bruno was great. I felt comfortable as soon as I walked into his office. He was able to see all my symptoms without me even telling him anything and he could even tell me things that I haven't even told my doctor, all by just looking into my eyes. He explained everything to me and in a way that I could understand it. He then went through what he recommended with a new eating plan as well as some tablets and powders. He said that within the first one to two months I would know if this was right for me. I cried a sign of relief that someone finally had given me some light at the end of the tunnel.

The eating plan was going to be tough, as I had to cut out anything sweet (I had been using sweet food especially jellybeans to give me energy and get through the day) as well as dairy foods and other foods such as white bread, coffee, alcohol and selected fruit, but if it meant that I would start to feel normal and back to my old self I would give it a go and follow the new eating plan.

Within the first week the eating plan was second nature, was easy to follow and my family joined me on it. I got into my habit of eating breakfast, morning tea, lunch, afternoon tea and dinner. I just could not believe how easy it was to change my habits. I noticed my energy levels had changed and I was feeling less tired by the middle of the first month. As the month went by I noticed less pain within my legs and muscles.

By the second month I noticed less of my hair falling out and I was starting to lose weight. Not only did my energy levels keep up with me but I was now sleeping through the whole night and not waking up fatigued and tired. I also noticed that the pain from the surgery was getting less and less frequent, my stress had also been reduced, and I felt more in control of my anxiety, feelings and emotions. It was also getting easier to eat the right foods and adapt foods when I went out to lunch or dinner. Life was looking good.

I have now been seeing Bruno for almost six months and I am still on The Marevich Way program and really enjoying the healthy eating. I am still on the tablets as well as on the powders which we are looking at slowly reducing. My energy levels are now high, I am sleeping through the night and have lost 35 kg. My hair is now back to normal and I only feel leg pain when I have been walking and running around a lot. I still have control of my stress levels and emotions. I guess you could say I'm now getting my mojo back as everyone has noticed a change within me and I am looking forward to a great new year with the new me.

I am so glad that Bruno was recommended to me. I have not looked back and I would recommend Bruno to everyone who wants to feel better and get their health and energy back.

Ingrid L.

COMMENTS: Ingrid is a good testimony to our liver's phenomenal innate ability to grow back and function again, often almost as though nothing much had happened, at least so in theory and assuming that the liver isn't subjected to the myriad of environmental and nutritional problems that almost everyone's liver has to deal with these days.

In reality, unfortunately much of what most people eat, drink, breathe, wear, absorb through their skin and hair – and also without any doubt think and dream i.e. their attitude to life – all of these can and do place extra burdens on an already very busy organ of the body. All of these burdens affect our liver's ability to work as well as it was meant to, and there is probably no clearer way of seeing this when, as in Ingrid's case, half or more of our liver has been removed. The liver will now have the extra duty of continuing to do all it is meant to do, with 'half of its staff away on leave', so to speak, and additionally, at the same time, regenerate, regrow and rebuilt itself.

Ingrid's poor liver was struggling to come back to normal after her operation. Using The Marevich Way, holistic dietary support and a supplements approach (yes including silymarin, of course), which has and will benefit practically everyone, whether with half or full liver, not only did Ingrid's health improve rapidly but also the other liver nutrients included in her program supported her liver for it to be able to go back to work relatively quickly and efficiently. When I last saw Ingrid face to face, she was as busy and flat out working as hard as a well-functioning liver, full of happiness and good intentions and I know that she still continues sticking to her healthy eating and a light maintenance program of supplements which her husband collects for her occasionally from our office to keep her liver happy. Love your Liver!

Many years ago, as a young naturopath, I was fortunate to have a brilliant mentor, a wise naturopath, great chiropractor and a real gentleman by the name of Robert Lucy. Robert has long passed away but some of his advice still resonates in my ears. He would often tell me, "If for all the people that come to see you with whatever problem they have, the only thing that you may manage to do is improve their liver, you will without questions have done their whole health a great service."

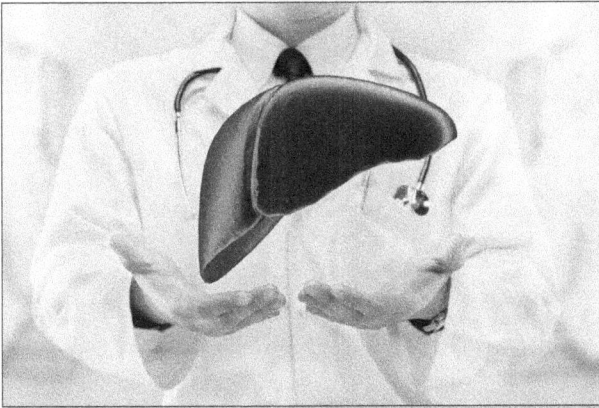

CHAPTER 5

Sure Way to Great Health

WELCOME TO
HEALTHY LIFE

ENJOY THE JOURNEY

CHAPTER 5

Sure Way to Great Health

Another very important condition which can have a massive impact upon our health and wellbeing, and influence our overall life in ways that we may not even begin to imagine, is hypoglycaemia. Like the digestive tract problems and their widespread prevalence discussed in the previous chapter, hypoglycaemia, or more precisely, reactive hypoglycaemia, is affecting the populations of the developed world in pandemic proportions and yet, when was the last time that your physician explained this to you?

Well, let me try to explain it you now as your awareness and understanding of this condition may reveal to you what you have been trying to understand about your health, and which has been eluding you for a long time. Understanding hypoglycaemia and knowing how to go about effectively treating the condition, unless you already do, may just end up being the single best thing that you have ever done or will ever do for yours and your family's health, as it has in fact been with tens of thousands of my patients over the past three decades.

Hypoglycaemia simply means low levels of sugar, or more precisely glucose, in the blood, following your ingestion of carbohydrates containing foods. But how can that be, don't carbohydrates raise your blood glucose? Yes they do, and that is where the problem begins, but let me first explain some important facts about this very important and very often problematic topic, carbohydrates.

The carbohydrates that we consume in our meals and snacks must get broken down by our digestive tracts into a much smaller molecule called glucose before they can be absorbed via our intestinal villi into our bloodstream and be delivered to the trillions of cells in our body which depend on glucose for their energy needs.

Carbohydrates are often referred to as simple or complex carbohydrates depending on how many molecules are stuck together to form the chain of molecules which becomes the carbohydrate.

Simple carbohydrates are made up of fewer molecules which do not take as long to digest and separate, and thus can be absorbed easily and quickly and can be a source of quick energy to our body when this is required.

The simplest of all commonly ingested carbohydrates is our common table sugar which consists of only two molecules, and is referred to as a disaccharide ('di-' as in consisting of two molecules).

The two simpler, one molecule substances (monosaccharides) that bond chemically together to form sugar, are called glucose and fructose. Fructose is also commonly found in fruit. A third monosaccharide is galactose which together with glucose makes up lactose, the disaccharide found in milk. For the sake of simplicity in the following examples, let us just remember that table sugar is made up of two simple molecules, glucose and fructose. Let us concentrate for the time being on the glucose molecule.

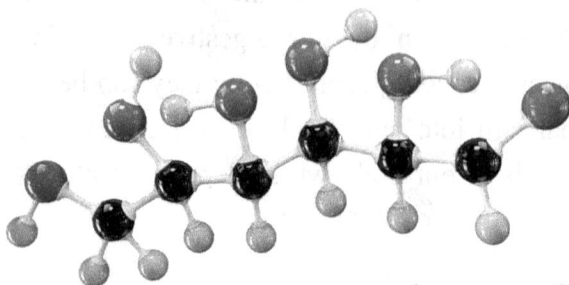

molecule of **Glucose**
C6H12O6
3D illustration

Common sugar is found in almost every food these days whether it has been added to sweeten the taste of the product or is naturally occurring – either way, whether you ingest it by eating an ice cream which will also probably contain many other not terribly natural or healthy ingredients, or in a glass of freshly squeezed natural orange juice, sugar is still sugar.

Sugar is therefore a very common, simple substance made up by only two molecules, which as you can imagine, does not require too long for our saliva and digestive tracts to separate into its two molecular components, glucose and fructose and to get absorbed into our blood.

Indeed a very quick digestive task for our bodies, when you consider that some of the more complex carbohydrates such as starches and cellulose found in some plants, roots and seeds (polysaccharides) are sometimes made up of long chains of tightly packed molecules that can add up to many thousands, and thus obviously require a lot longer to digest and absorb into our bloodstream than do soft drinks, biscuits or cakes.

Case History no. 12 – Peta's personal testimonial.

After suffering from abnormally heavy periods (menorrhagia) and severe endometriosis for over 20 years, a friend highly recommended I make an appointment with Bruno. Despite having seen countless doctors, specialists and naturopaths, I was hopeful Bruno could assist as I had seen my friend's health greatly improve in a short timeframe under Bruno's care. I am eternally grateful to my friend for recommending such a great naturopath to assist me on my path to great health.

From the onset, Bruno was extremely caring, helpful, knowledgeable and compassionate. Bruno listened to my every word and asked many questions to confirm what he was seeing in my eyes and from my body in general. Bruno recommended a specific diet in conjunction with tablets appropriate for my health issues. Bruno carefully explained what foods I had to eliminate and why. I greatly appreciated Bruno explaining technical health information in an easy to understand way.

Due to the severity of my conditions, it took about four months before I started to feel human again. I felt better than I had in 30 years. My periods were regular and only lasted five days (previously, I had bled very heavily for six months straight). For the first time in 20 years, my iron levels were consistently good and I didn't need weekly iron injections or blood transfusions. I found I became very sensitive to foods I had eliminated which made it difficult to eat out with friends but I was determined to look after myself. I tried very hard to resist friend's food temptations. Due to work stresses, I sometimes had bad weeks not taking the recommended tablets and not eating appropriately. Bruno was always incredibly positive, helpful and caring, getting me back on track.

Work pressure resulted in poor quality of sleep. Bruno tweaked my tablets and food and I finally started getting quality sleep. I was finally waking up rested and ready to tackle the day.

After being under Bruno's care for about 12 months, I decided to move away from Sydney. I was very concerned about continuing on my wellness path without regular naturopath appointments with Bruno. I enquired whether I could come and see Bruno every few months as I wanted to continue under his care. No problem is ever too big for Bruno – he treats patients all over the world so we could have appointments via phone and I could order my tablets from him.

Due to stress from the move, I fell back into old and bad eating habits. Bruno helped get me back on track. After a few months, I developed extremely bad psoriasis on my scalp. It was extremely sore and I found it very difficult to touch or comb my hair. My hair was falling out in large clumps. I thought it was due to Brisbane's unusually hot and humid summer. I sought assistance from doctors and specialists and I was given antibiotics and told to apply cream regularly and that it would clear up when the weather cooled down. Six months later, the weather had cooled down but my psoriasis had spread to my ears and nostrils.

In desperation, I sought Bruno's assistance. I wish I had contacted him months earlier! Within a few weeks the psoriasis had greatly improved and within a few months, it had completely cleared up. Even though this consultation was over the phone, Bruno immediately knew what was causing the psoriasis and what I needed to do to restore good health. I cannot thank Bruno enough for his invaluable assistance, guidance, care and patience while I have been under his care. Do not hesitate, call Bruno today!

Peta E.

COMMENTS: Peta's long debilitating symptoms (mainly hormonal, food sensitivities, psoriasis and low iron count) were resolved without any direct hormonal nor skin interventions, but rather by balancing her sugar metabolism and digestive issues – of which Peta, like most people, was largely unaware – and with the use of our diet and our supplements, The Marevich Way, to help these causative problems.

From my experience, together with the intestinal absorption conditions discussed in the previous chapter, it is my professional opinion that these two conditions combine to either directly or indirectly cause the overwhelmingly large number of fatigue, pain, all kinds of disease, suffering and premature deaths suffered in our world today. Big assumptions or conclusion you may think.

When I first started observing the strange but vast effects that this condition was having with our patients many years ago, hypoglycaemia was, and it kind of still is, considered by medicine mainly as a glucose low in our blood, most commonly seen with diabetics who have taken an excessive amount of medicinal insulin to lower the high blood glucose levels that occur with people who suffer with diabetes. Their blood's glucose tends to raise too high (hyperglycaemia) for several possible reasons, but mostly because their pancreases are no longer producing as much insulin as they should and also their cells have become desensitised to what insulin should do, which is to allow the glucose in the blood to enter inside these living cells that make up our bodies.

These days science is far more aware that there are also other causes apart from excessive medicinal insulin that will cause the blood sugar to become unstable and fall more rapidly that it should. The condition has been given names such as reactive hypoglycaemia, low blood sugar, insulin resistance or metabolic syndrome. They are really all one and the same problem.

The glucose in our blood can be easily determined even at home with a finger prick and an electronic blood glucose meter, which can be purchased relatively inexpensively in pharmacies by anyone, thus making remaining ignorant of this condition less necessary.

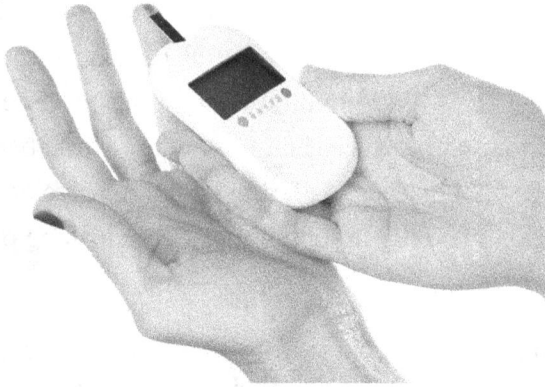

Even then, a large percentage of the world's population is unaware of the fact that they are diabetic, despite doctors and nutritionists having been raising awareness and concerns about this condition for decades now. Quite rightly so, that they would raise it, as modern medicine at the moment is clearly losing the fight against type 2 diabetes, also referred to as adult onset diabetes, and the vast multitude of other problems, suffering and mortality it causes, including at least doubling the risk of early death.

As at 2015, International Diabetes Federation stated that there are approximately 415 million adult diabetics in the world, one out of every 11 people.

In Australia, according to the same diabetes monitoring body, there were some 1.2 million diabetics known and registered (one out of every 20 Australians). Current estimates are that, in addition to the

1.2 million diabetics, there are another four million 'pre-diabetic' in Australia, (one out of every six Australians, whether young or old).

> Statistics indicate 280 people develop diabetes every day in Australia, that's one every five minutes!

Unfortunately the real figures are almost certainly far more sinister, as it is thought that the real total numbers of diabetics in the world could be anywhere between 20% to 50% higher when taking into account large numbers of undiagnosed people who are diabetic but they don't know it. The planet's major monitoring agency, the Centers for Disease Control (CDC) has declared diabetes as an epidemic and predicts that *"without major changes, as many as 1 in 3 (33%) US adults could have diabetes by 2050"*.

There are no reliable estimates as to how many people are hypoglycaemic, which could be defined as the 'pre-pre-diabetic' stage, in Australia or anywhere in the world. One will have been pre-diabetic before having become diabetic. Whilst not every hypoglycaemic will necessary become pre-diabetic and not every pre-diabetic will develop diabetes, it is safe to assume that every diabetic was once pre-diabetic and hypoglycaemic before that.

Whilst there is some statistical consolation that not every hypoglycaemic will become pre-diabetic and not every pre-diabetic will progress to diabetes, it is certainly nothing to be too relaxed about.

For every registered diabetic person in the previously mentioned statistics, the figures show that there are at least 2.5 other pre-diabetic people waiting to become diabetic. My personal clinical estimates, developed by observation of tens of thousands of my patients' reactions to different diets and supplements, is that for every pre-diabetic person there are, conservatively, at least three people whose health problems are, at one level or another. being directly affected by hypoglycaemia.

Case Study no. 13– Andrew's personal testimonial.

Some ten years ago my health was suffering. I was overweight with high insulin levels and given the recent loss of a family member, was also depressed. I went to my local GP and went on a mainstream antidepressant. The side effects were enormous, including driving to work and nearly falling asleep at the wheel one day. The GP advised a stimulant drug to stay awake. I was not keen to take further drugs and sensed that I was spiralling downwards with failed diets. Not knowing what to do I thought a naturopath was worth a try and discovered Bruno.

I was sceptical at first but he helped me get off the antidepressants and go on a natural alternative with no side effects. Through a complete change in diet and supplement program I lost weight, improved cholesterol and my sense of wellbeing also improved significantly. Type 2 diabetes was no longer a threat. Prior to starting the program Bruno said that blood test results would change and improve and after being on the program they did as expected.

I was amazed and haven't looked back since. I know more now about what foods to avoid and what to include and the importance of exercise. There is so much misinformation out there but now I am more educated and discerning. I am a real life example of health success in a modern world. Thanks Bruno.

Andrew C.

COMMENTS: Andrew also suffered with a large variety of food intolerances and sensitivities when he first came to see me. He had been on numerous diet programs to try and control these problems and their debilitating effects but with only limited success. Helping improve Andrew's blood-sugar metabolism and thus serotonin levels by following The Marevich Way helped him get off the medicines that were not really achieving this for him and avoid their strong side effects. The healing and stabilising of the digestive tract helped improve his immune system and, yes, he has been quite successful and continues to take good care of his health.

These figures add up to at least 12 million hypoglycaemic in Australia. This is, at least, every second person! Every second person in Australia and therefore almost certainly in most of the rest of world, suffering with an undiagnosed condition which is likely to be already contributing to a multitude of other clinical or subclinical conditions going undiagnosed, and thus unhelped by the health system. This also means that more likely than not, most people who have been diagnosed with a health condition have most likely received a diagnosis and prescribed with medicinal drugs primarily based on their symptoms, rather than the true causative factors, in which poor intestinal permeability and reactive hypoglycaemia are almost certainly playing a leading role. This further means that the patients' real causative problems have been left untreated and are thus most likely still slowly brewing in the background to develop into something more serious like perhaps, eventually, diabetes but perhaps even something worse.

> Unfortunately, the real cause of most illnesses will never get official diagnosed nor recognised as having been originated or aided in their progress by hypoglycaemia nor pre-diabetes.

And even if these conditions are picked up via blood tests done to determine the cause of their illness, they may only get referred to as just one more, unrelated problem with little or no relationship to the patients' official condition or illness

The most common causes of death are cardiovascular diseases and cancers. These may not have been necessarily caused directly by hypoglycaemia or pre-diabetes in every case. However, almost certainly they would have been made worse, further complicated, and their recovery or remission hindered, slowed down and perhaps even blocked by one of these two glucose metabolism conditions which the overwhelming percentage of the world is affected by.

The patient will have been instead, whilst fighting to get better, more likely been diagnosed by their doctor with a condition that more reflects their symptoms and have either been prescribed painkillers, blood pressure medication, cholesterol lowering drugs, anti-inflammatories, antacids, hormonal replacements, steroids, heart medicines, antibiotics or worse, anticancer drugs. Again, these drugs may be necessary for some patients with an advanced illness and resulting poor overall general health. Embarking on a "natural-medicines-only" treatment may at this advanced stage be too slow or risky. The dangerous side effects of the drugs may be a lesser risk than not taking them at all.

Let us clarify how our blood sugar or glucose should ideally behave and what often goes wrong. At fasting, before having any food in the morning, blood glucose level is considered normal, according to the recommended range figures printed on most blood test, if it reads somewhere between 3.5 to 5.5 mmol/L (millimoles of glucose in every one litre of blood). Different pathology laboratories and different countries may use a slightly different range such as 4.0 to 6.0. Also, mmol/L is a form of measurement used in Australia and many other parts of the world, such as parts of Europe and Asia, whereas other countries such as the US use mg/dL instead (milligrams of glucose in a decilitre of blood) just to make things a little more interesting. It is not hard though to convert mmol/L to mg/dL. Just multiply by 18 (i.e. 4 mmol/L x 18= 72 mg/dL and 6 mmol/L x 18= 108 mg/dL).

At the testing laboratory, if your fasting blood glucose is higher than the recommend high level (6.1mmol/L or higher) and, after having been given 75 g of glucose to drink and after waiting two more hours, the reading is now above 11 mmol/L then you will generally be officially declared as a type 2 diabetic and probably be prescribed drugs and hopefully nutritional and exercise advice to try and improve your readings.

Again, quite rightly so because the problems associated with diabetes can be quite serious and should of course be avoided. Apart from probably simply making one's life statistically shorter than the average population as well as less enjoyable, diabetics are the most common victims of kidney failure, lower limb amputation and adult blindness.

Other serious concerns are nerve damage, heart disease and stroke, the world's biggest killers. Fortunately adult onset diabetes is called so because it can take many years, 20, 30 or even more to slowly develop before one is diagnosed accordingly, Having said that, the average age of discovering that one is now officially diabetic has been alarmingly coming down over the last few years. The average estimated age for the onset of adult diabetes is 54 to 55 years old. Young ones are however not completely risk free, as it is also estimated that 12 out of 100,000 people will develop adult onset diabetes much earlier with the average age of this group being only 14 years young! Worrying figures? Of course.

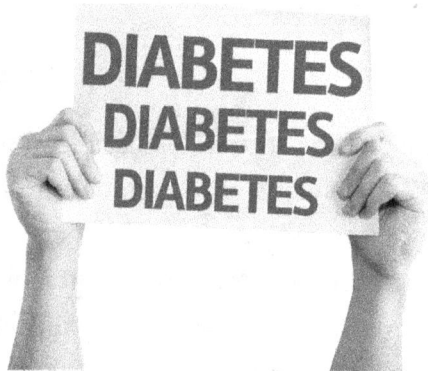

However, even though there is the risk that one day in the not too distant future this condition could also become a teenagers and perhaps even a childhood condition, at least for the moment we know that in most cases one has many years before its official diagnosis to try and do something about it.

How? Well we all know that prevention is better than cure but the difficult part is that it is generally not so easy to work hard at eating healthy, deprive ourselves of foods and drinks to which the world as a whole is addicted, to try prevent a condition that you may never ever develop and miss out on all the fun. After all, your last blood test may actually have shown your fasting blood glucose levels to be well within the goal posts shown on the report and there is a chance that it may not deviate too greatly as time goes on and as you age. At least this is probably how most of us rationalise.

Case Study no. 14 – Stephanie's personal testimonial.

With Bruno's help, in the last 18 months I have been able to lose 50 kgs, clear my skin and rebalance my whole body. My whole life has changed thanks to Bruno's well-balanced approach to health.

I have struggled all my life with my weight and many doctors have told me that to lose weight would be almost impossible due to hormonal imbalances, however, with Bruno's supplements, he has been able to improve my hormone imbalance and help me drop nearly six dress sizes. I have also been able to subdue the anxiety and depression I suffered before. Every appointment he monitors closely what the whole body is doing and suggests adjustments in diet/supplements to make sure everything in the body is healthy.

I have never felt healthier, fitter or been as slim in my entire life and I know I owe it all to Bruno and his amazing naturopathy knowledge and skills. It's set me up for the rest of my life to never want to go back to the way I was and also being able to maintain all that has been accomplished.

Stephanie D.

COMMENTS: Stephanie's dogged determination to get rid of her unwanted weight was made a lot easier by her strict compliance to The Marevich Way program of correct eating and supplements. Her regular exercise routine also contributed greatly to her fantastic results. Improving her sugar metabolism made this great effort more possible as hypoglycaemia will make it almost impossible to control ones serotonin, leptin and dopamine hormones making the addiction to sugars very difficult to break. This then perpetuates the "try to diet" followed by hunger, frustration, boredom and depression followed by seeking relief by overindulging in the wrong foods again followed by guilt and putting on more weight and eventually the decision to go back to the diet again, making the cycle almost impossible to break. One of the most common expression of gratitude that we hear from many patients isn't "thank you for getting rid of my migraines" or "thank you for giving me a perfect skin" (results which by the way we have a great deal of success with), but instead "thank you for helping me remove the shackles that had me enslaved to sugar. These days I no longer need it and I can decide what I want to do, no different than eating a tomato or a cucumber". By taking these actions during a relatively young age Stephanie has very importantly reduced her statistical chances of diabetes and thus other possibly serious conditions in the future.

What if I told you that the probability of diabetes can actually be determined way, way before you are 54 or 55 years old in most people? And not only by looking at your fasting sugar levels as these may take many years to creep up above the recommended figures.

It can even be determined a lot earlier than when first hearing from a good doctor that your blood glucose, although within the range, is beginning to creep too close for comfort to the high range and starts to suspect a pre-diabetic condition. Yes, although diagnosing pre-diabetes is still better than having waited to find out that your blood glucose is skyrocketing and you have been diabetic for who knows how many years, even the event of pre-diabetes could have been foreseen many years before. If one is pre-diabetic, they are not just outside the periphery of a war zone, they are already where bombs are being dropped and already at a high risk of being injured by the same projectiles as the ones intended for those in the middle of the conflict.

Whilst the fasting glucose level is one indicator of impaired blood glucose metabolism, what your glucose does after you have had your first meal and broken your fast is also vitally important but unfortunately very disregarded and under-monitored by most health professionals.

Let us say for the sake of the example that you are still a long way away from the statistical age of onset of diabetes, 54 to 55 years old. Let us say that you are somewhere between 18 and 50 years of age and your fasting glucose is somewhere well within the required 4 to 6 mmol/L , say a very good level of 5. Let us say that you had a blood test only because you like to keep a check on your health or because you have one of the many conditions that drive people to see doctors, and had a general blood test done to gather further information to help identify the source of your condition. It could be as simple as not feeling so well or energetic lately, suffering with the occasional headache or some other pain or an irregular hormonal system down to being afflicted with another already identified condition such as chronic fatigue, fibromyalgia, blood pressure, high cholesterol levels etc. etc.

It is almost certain that with a fasting blood glucose level of 5, your physician would not even bother to suspect that there may be anything untoward with your blood glucose. Unfortunately, as we will see, this is a flawed assumption and a dangerous one at that because, to a trained physician, your other health problems or the reason that you went to see him should raise suspicions that the fasting level may not be completely indicative of what your glucose metabolism is up to.

You see, even though your fasting glucose may be a very comfortable 5, the blood glucose does not remain like that for the rest of the day. Blood glucose goes up and down the whole day depending on when and what you are eating and drinking, your exercising habits or lack thereof and how hard you are making your adrenal glands work.

After say breakfast, from a normal 5 mmol/L, the glucose levels will go up, depending on what you are eating and how much sugar or carbohydrates are in your breakfast to anywhere between 7 to 8 mmol/L and then it should gradually over the next five to six hours glide back down to the starting, pre-breakfast fasting level of 5 using this example. Unfortunately these days, fewer and fewer people seem to fit this pattern.

> Most blood glucose tests of non-diabetic patients these days reveal blood glucose levels that rise pretty much as expected but fall down much more rapidly than desirable.

It is not unusual to see patients who undertake the standard two hour glucose tolerance test (GTT) at a laboratory where their fasting blood glucose is measured first upon their arrival, are then given a drink containing 75 grams of glucose, and then over the next two hours have their blood glucose tested hourly again, that they have in fact already returned to fasting, some three or four hours earlier than they should have. Some will have even returned to fasting earlier than the two hours after drinking the glucose, and their blood glucose will actually have dropped below the 5 mmol/L used in our example, at times as low as 3.5 mmol/L or even lower. They will generally know it because they will not be quite feeling completely like "they are there" and may even at times take several hours to recover. Years ago, doctors would quite regularly request a five hours glucose tolerance test (GTT) which would reveal a lot more information regarding how their patient's body handled glucose.

Today's two hours test is mainly performed to see whether you are actually diabetic as yet or not quite, in which case you may be asked to come back and have it checked again in a few more months, to see whether your train has arrived at the station as yet or not.

This rapid fall of blood sugar in every day's life does not go unnoticed by most people. It is often experienced following a carbohydrate loaded breakfast as is quite common these days. Breakfast cereals with low fat milk and god forbid a few spoons of sugar, followed by a glass of fruit juice or a cup of coffee, is as bad as it gets. The glucose will be absorbed so quickly in the blood that its count will skyrocket, often as much as the energy will. All this quick energy, without having to wake up the stomach and the liver who are still recovering from last night's dinner, from their slumber.

Quick energy, and almost baby food not requiring any real effort from our already lazy digestive tract – what could appear to be better? Unfortunately the quick raise of our glucose comes at a price. Because this kind of eating style, rich in carbohydrates, may have been our way of feeding our bodies for a number of years already, the cells in our body no longer absorb the sugar as well and as fast as they should from our blood. This causes our pancreas to have to release more and more insulin to stimulate our cells to absorb the glucose. More information about this in the next few pages. For now, enough to say that the excessive build-up of insulin can eventually cause the glucose to become absorbed too quickly from the blood into our cells, causing it to fall sharply, often below fasting levels within a couple of hours.

At that stage the brain that, although weighing only about 2% of our body's total weight actually uses some 50 to 70% of the glucose in our blood, will begin to make it very clear that if it is expected to work, it wants you to procure some more sugar, and it usually wants it now!

This will cause most people around about morning tea time to go for a cup of tea or coffee with a biscuit or perhaps a fruit, which will just bring the blood glucose rapidly back to where it was before, either because of the ingested sugar or the adrenal stimulation.

Others, whose digestive tract is just beginning to recover from the large or late dinner last night, will not feel in the mood for any foods despite their brain's supplications. In that case, the brain will actually take over and instruct the adrenal glands to release adrenaline. Adrenaline has several functions and one of those is to convince our liver, the container of stored glucose in the form of glycogen, to convert it back to glucose an release it into the bloodstream. So, some people will have a cup of tea or coffee for morning tea and others who don't, will have instead adrenaline and glucose donated by their liver. Either way, food or no food, the sugar level will rise again and give us another leg-up to continue with our brain and muscular activities for a few more hours.

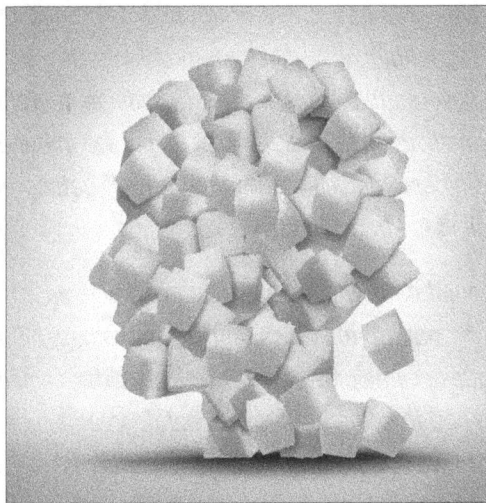

It is often after lunch, commonly between 1.00 pm and 3.00 pm that what seemed a good idea and helpful with our energy and focus in the morning no longer now appears to be so. Some people will feel tired, some will feel a brain fog and find it hard to concentrate or motivate. Others have learned that another good cup of coffee will give them the final energy boost required to see the working day out. Others, with more determination and perhaps also greater adrenal storage to help them transit through the rest of the afternoon will still manage to squeeze those last few drops of adrenaline through sheer motivation and desire to accomplish their day's work. They will not notice until the day's work has ended, have come back home and the motivational carrot or need to push themselves has been removed, that they are pretty bankrupt as far as energy is concerned.

Case Study no. 15– Nadine's personal testimonial.

My first migraine was at the age of ten and so started my long battle with migraines, fatigue and digestive problems. In '98 I injured my spine and discovered that I was allergic to codeine, morphine and other mainstream medications. This led me to pursue natural medicine. I started with Chinese medicine but found myself getting migraines just from the smell of the herbs in the clinic.

I eventually found naturopathic treatment and was so impressed that I started to study natural therapies, but my migraines, all over the body pain and fatigue became unbearable, to the point that I could not continue studying, so I had to settle for a nutritional degree instead. At this point I believed that I was in the heart of natural therapies and was living the lifestyle. Unfortunately I was so fatigued that I could only manage to be awake for three to four hours a day. My legs would feel like they were bags of sand and I struggled to stand and walk.

Then I was told about Bruno Marevich at Australian Naturopathics. I agreed to start on Bruno's products and give The Marevich Way treatment protocol my best.

I immediately felt different.

At that time, being still a newly graduated nutritionist I researched all of Bruno's designed own supplements and tried to understand why these products made me feel better than all the other top of the line 'Practitioner Only Products' which I had taken for many years.

The answer is that a Bruno has stuck to the fundamentals of naturopathic philosophy and has managed to create a combination of products that make it easier for the client/patient to take. A basic seven products rather than the 26 or more that I had been using prior to visiting Bruno.

I currently may get a migraine three or four times a year, rather than weekly. I was also able to lose weight despite my back pain and chronic fatigue. My fatigue and pain are still work in progress and I cannot deny that whatever adjustment or addition of vitamins Bruno has made has been truly spot on for my progress.

The support and mentoring that I have received from Bruno has not only helped me and the people that I have referred to Bruno, but also in my clinic with my own clients whom I treat and get great results with by following The Marevich Way. Thank you Bruno.

Nadine A.

COMMENTS: There is nothing like trusting so much on the treatment protocol that you are following for yourself, as Nadine does, that you also want to help your own patients and family with the same products and protocol. There are not many other greater indicators or reassurances of a product's benefits that a patient could receive than that. Next time you see a health practitioner ask if they are also on the same health gaining or disease prevention program and products as they are recommending for you. If the answer is yes, you may probably not be able to be in better hands.

Nadine is also very open with declaring that her present health, particularly fatigue and pains are still not as good as what she would like them to be, despite no lack of time and effort having been spared to ameliorate them.

Nadine's case study is a useful one because it is a little different to almost every other one in the book, apart from perhaps Pam's case study number 17. The moral of the story is that despite every patient I have ever placed on The Marevich Way protocol having improved, the great majority many times exceeding even my or their own expectations, for some – fortunately a very small minority – the improvements are there but not as much as we would have liked. Again, the overall number of these patients can probably be counted on the fingers of my and perhaps your hands only. Not bad out of tens of thousands, considering that even these few patients still happily admit to feeling better than before. I never wanted the book to include the case histories of the most successful patients only, but a fair cross-section that will give the reader a better and more realistic view of the benefits of natural medicine. Not everyone gets fixed 'forever and on the spot' although it often seems that way. After all we are all surrounded by ongoing environmental stresses which not everyone will ever be capable of dealing with equally as well. Also, health should not only be viewed as a destination. It is indeed a journey. Getting well is not always a guarantee that we will remain that way forever. Anything that can be repaired can also be broken again unless we continue to care for it. Good news just on hand from Nadine, almost as my completed manuscript for this book is about to be handed over to the publisher for printing, is that the new trials we have made with the balancing of Nadine's supplements appear to be giving her even better results.

Energy, in biochemical terms, is the fuel that keeps us going and in health terms, energy is the "currency for healing". No fuel in the car, the engine shuts down. Poor or no energy in our body, poor or no healing nor repair. When my patients come back for their follow-up visit, apart from the usual questions on how they are handling the program that I have put them on, the most important question I can ask them is how their energy is going.

Regardless as to why they have come to see me in the first instance, heart problems, blood pressure, migraines, etc., etc., their energy status is always the most important indicator to me as to how they are improving metabolically and how well they may be on their journey of healing and recovery.

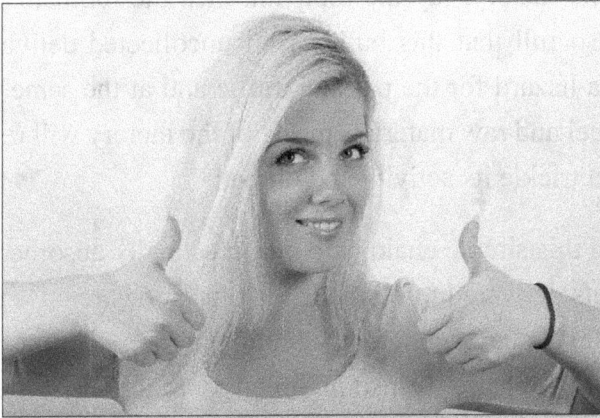

Let's examine a little more how all of this actually works, and why it happens in the way that I have just explained.

Once the glucose from our simple or complex carbohydrate foods has been digested into glucose and absorbed into our bloodstream, this is just the beginning of our body's responses which are defined as our carbohydrate metabolism.

Consider the blood circulation as a highway that delivers all of our nutrients including glucose to the many trillions of living cells all over our body in every organ, muscle and tissue, head to toes. The nutrients therefore do not really belong in the blood, they are meant to be transported inside of the cells. The blood circulation therefore delivers the raw materials and fuel absorbed from the intestines into the many trillions of microscopic but complex factories, our cells.

Usually these nutrients, once delivered to the front step of the factory, require help – "forklift trucks or conveyor belts" to take them inside the factory for specialised processing depending on what they are meant to be used for. If they are not brought in from outside the factory, say the footpath, then the footpath will soon become so full that this build-up of uncollected deliveries may become a hazard for the passing traffic and at the same time, the lack of fuel and raw materials inside of the factory will reduce and bring to a trickle its activity and output.

Applying this simple analogy to our intestinally absorbed glucose which gets delivered to our cells via our bloodstream – when our glucose levels have gone higher following a meal, our pancreas, senses it and release its insulin directly into the bloodstream. The major job that this hormone, insulin, needs to accomplish is to give instructions to our cells to absorb the glucose in the blood for their internal processing into energy, i.e. open wide the front door of the factory and empower the forklift trucks and conveyor belts to get the deliveries off the front footpath and inside the factory.

Insulin achieves this by binding itself on its receptor found on the membrane that surrounds and encapsulates our cells. This begins a series of protein activation cascades which allow the glucose to enter our cells from the blood.

Insulin is the key that opens the door of the factory to allow the glucose piled up on the front footpath to be transported into the factory.

If the pancreas is incapable of producing enough insulin or the cells have become desensitised and require greater amounts of insulin, the glucose may not get absorbed by the cells for use as fuel, and remains in our blood where its levels increase to heights which can be damaging to various organs and their functions.

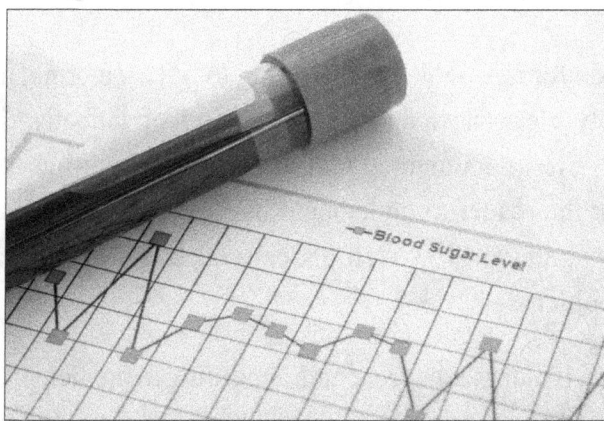

As explained earlier, fortunately, in adult onset diabetes, as the name suggests, the condition does not occur overnight. It is a long and laborious task lasting many years of us consuming sugar containing foods, expecting our pancreas to work all sorts of hours, every time we feel like a snack, and for the pancreas to eventually decide that it has worked more hours than it was at first employed to work and is now getting tired and is no longer capable of withstanding the demands and long hours it could when it was young. The combination of reduced insulin being released by our pancreas into our blood and cells which actually demand even more insulin than they used to is the basis of the process known as adult onset diabetes.

Nothing terribly new in any of the above explanations for the most common causes of diabetes. Most common because there are always other factors that may affect the process such as genetic predispositions, body weight factors, exercise, other hormonal factors, etc., and modern medicine is quite well aware, in deep scientific detail, of how this all works as well as to what the risk factors for diabetes are.

The reason for this book endeavouring to impart a basic, hopefully reasonably clear view and understanding of diabetes, is to use this fairly well documented and understood condition to make it easier for the reader to understand hypoglycaemia, an even more widespread and yet less well understood and medically accepted health problem.

Therefore, if diabetes has reached, according to medicine, epidemic levels, hypoglycaemia can then be compared, in numbers, to the pandemic bubonic plague that decimated Europe in the fourteenth century.

An estimated half of the world's population is at this earlier-than-pre-diabetic, hypoglycaemic stage. The chances are quite strong, as statistics imply at the moment, that hypoglycaemia will develop into pre-diabetes and then into diabetes.

> The CDC predicts that *"1 in 3 could have diabetes by 2050 unless major changes happen"*.

As explained, just because it develops earlier than pre-diabetes, hypoglycaemia should not be mistakenly thought of as just a minor problem that may never develop into anything more serious than the occasional tiredness or mid-afternoon yawn. Most patients that come to see me and other health care professionals will rarely, if ever, come because they know or suspect that they may be hypoglycaemic. I can count on the fingers of one hand the number of patients I have ever seen who came into our clinic, sat in front of me and said words to this effect "the reason for coming to see you today is that I am hypoglycaemic and I need your help to better manage this condition".

The reason for patients visiting us will normally be because they either:

- Have not been able to be diagnosed by medicine as to the reason for their condition, or are not satisfied with the diagnosis.

- Have been diagnosed correctly by their doctor with one of a many common or not so common chronic medical conditions and would prefer not to take drugs for the longer term if possible as they are concerned by their known and unknown side effects.

- Have been diagnosed and also treated for various lengths of time and by several physicians but have not been seeing satisfactory improvements.

- Have been recommended to us by one of the many caring doctors who these days understand that the prolonged use of drugs alone may not necessarily be in the patient's best health interest.

- Or, they are not aware of any health problems and want to keep it that way as *"prevention is better that cure"*.

And yet, the common story which they inevitably reveal when I dig deep and the patient expresses how they really feel beyond what they simply think they should say that fits their current medical diagnosis, inevitably almost always points to hypoglycaemia being associated with the condition.

The list of symptoms that hypoglycaemia may produce is practically longer than one's arm, and includes a surprisingly large variety of problems, including tiredness, headaches, dizziness, depressions, mood swings, irritability, insomnia, digestive disturbances, phobias, lack of sex drive, limited attention span, muscle and joint pains, various forms of addictions and hyperactivity and bedwetting in children. Almost all hypoglycaemic also suffer with candidiasis, a condition which indicates an overgrowth of the yeast candida in the gastrointestinal tract and is a potent source of allergies such as asthma.

> In fact hypoglycaemia has been called
> "the mimic of all diseases".

When we consider that in 1920 the average person consumed 11 kilograms of sugar per annum and in 1990 that had spiralled to

120 kilograms, it is perhaps not difficult to see why so many suffer with symptoms from sugar metabolism problems.

Patients at our clinic are also assessed for sugar metabolism imbalances with the help of Eye Diagnosis (an advanced form of iridology) and at times additional glucose tolerance tests are obtained. They are treated holistically and often begin to report dramatic improvement to their symptoms, including much increased vitality within a few short weeks – often in days and at times practically the day after.

But it does not end there, because as stated earlier, energy is the currency for healing. As the blood-sugar level improves with the correct diet and supplements, the original problem that brought them to the clinic also improves. A better sugar metabolism helps the body get healthier. A healthy body can take care of any problems better and more easily than a body that is not healthy and is lacking in energy.

Hypoglycaemia can therefore be improved by modifying our diets and assisting with natural supplements to help improve our metabolism. At our clinic, we are strong advocates of a hypoglycaemic diet for almost every patient we see and we continually see patients achieve high energy and optimum health by improving their body's blood-sugar metabolism.

Patients will regularly report within a few short weeks that they have better energy morning to night, sleep more deeply all night long and get up in the morning feeling refreshed and, for the first time they remember, feeling eager to get out of bed and start the day invigorated and motivated. The changes that we often see in people's lives are quite phenomenal as they no longer feel physically and mentally weighed down – they sense that their bodies are healing and feel even more encouraged when, visiting their doctors, they get told "I don't know what you are doing, but whatever it is, it is working so keep on doing it".

Case Study no. 16 – Glynis' personal testimonial.

After a motor vehicle accident in 2001. I started using painkillers and anti-inflammatory tablets almost daily for back pain. Later, I moved on to the 'heavy' painkillers and increased the dosages of the painkiller and the anti-inflammatory, and all this under the supervision of a neurosurgeon.

I also started to take sleeping tablets and when the Drs decided not to prescribe them any longer, I was already addicted. This went on for seven years and in 2008, I collapsed and was hospitalised. I had to have surgery on my spine, and the neurosurgeon informed me that the operation would only be a 'pain reliever' for two years, and I would need more than one operation on my spine and neck to sort out my problems. I had the surgery and after a long recovery, the pain was back, and so, I started the cycle all over again, and more tablets were added to the list, including tablets for anxiety, depression, and muscle relaxants.

One day, I told a friend how sick the medication made me feel and the horrible side effects that the medication had caused. Among other things: migraines, headaches, gastro and liver problems, rapid weight gain, dry mouth, insomnia, palpitations, sweats, tiredness, ulcers and high blood pressure. She advised me to see a naturopath, whom I contacted immediately out of sheer desperation.

The first visit with Bruno Marevich will always be stuck in my mind. He immediately diagnosed most of my health problems just by looking into

---

my eyes. I was in awe that his diagnosis was so accurate without having told him what was wrong with me, but I very much doubted when he told me that I would feel like a new person after his program. In my mind I replied "yeah right".

I started a six months program using the natural products and supplements prescribed by him, and also weekly Myorthotics sessions, whilst I continued to take the supplements prescribed by Bruno. Under his guidance, after two months I was able to stop taking the antidepressants and sleeping tables and after another month, I stopped taking all other prescription medication. I currently only take the supplements and products that Bruno prescribed. I don't need the prescribed medication because I am pain free and feel like a new person.

His products are all natural and thus did not cause me any side effects. Rather, they reversed all the bad side effects of my prescribed medicines. I have been pain free for months, sleeping well, lost weight, my cholesterol and sugar levels are down and most of all I can actually enjoy my life. I have started walking four kilometres three times a week. something which I have not been able to do for 13 years!!

Bruno has supported me and guided me through this program, The Marevich Way, unlike my doctors who could not have cared less. He also showed a personal interest in my wellbeing and guided me step by step through the program. Thank you for your help Bruno Marevich, the journey was well worth it!!! I will continue on this path as long as possible.

Glynis D.

COMMENTS: Glynis' reaction to the drugs employed to bring some relief to the consequences of her motor vehicle accident and the surgery unfortunately also brought a long number of side effects. After identifying Glynis' poor digestion and absorption of food and nutrient issues in her stomach and intestines, her sugar metabolism imbalances, and the way that these were combining to aggravate her spinal condition, we had already started Glynis on her way to recovery. The right diet and supplements quickly started to work at correcting her overall state of health, I refer to it as "putting the body back into a healing mode". Because a healthy body takes care of everything better than one that is not healthy, together with the help of Myorthotics treatments (gentle muscle and ligaments support technique) Glynis' bad back symptoms, the major concern that brought her to the clinic, began to rapidly improve. Soon, a person who had been in almost constant chronic pain for many years and who other experts could not help, was capable of enjoying long walks and exercise which in turn assisted with her weight and even further back stabilisation.

The connection between the gut and the sugar level, and other seemingly unrelated parts of the body like the spine is rarely seen as significant or as asset for healing by modern medicine. This is partly understandable if we consider this statement with medical eyes only. Whilst not impossible, trying to find a reasonable, plausible and convincing, either biochemical, neurological or hormonal connection that could explain to a team of scientists or doctors the reasons for Glynis' massive improvements, would not be so easy. Not so easy, because not everything that happens in the body – its miraculous ability for healing, the additional benefits of a mind that is no longer depressed due to fluctuations of sugar related hormones and neurotransmitters and a patient who is now beginning to see a light at the end of a long and painful tunnel – can be explained by simple anatomy, physiology and biochemistry and science. At least not so well, not right now anyway.

CHAPTER 6

Health's Four Other Cornerstones

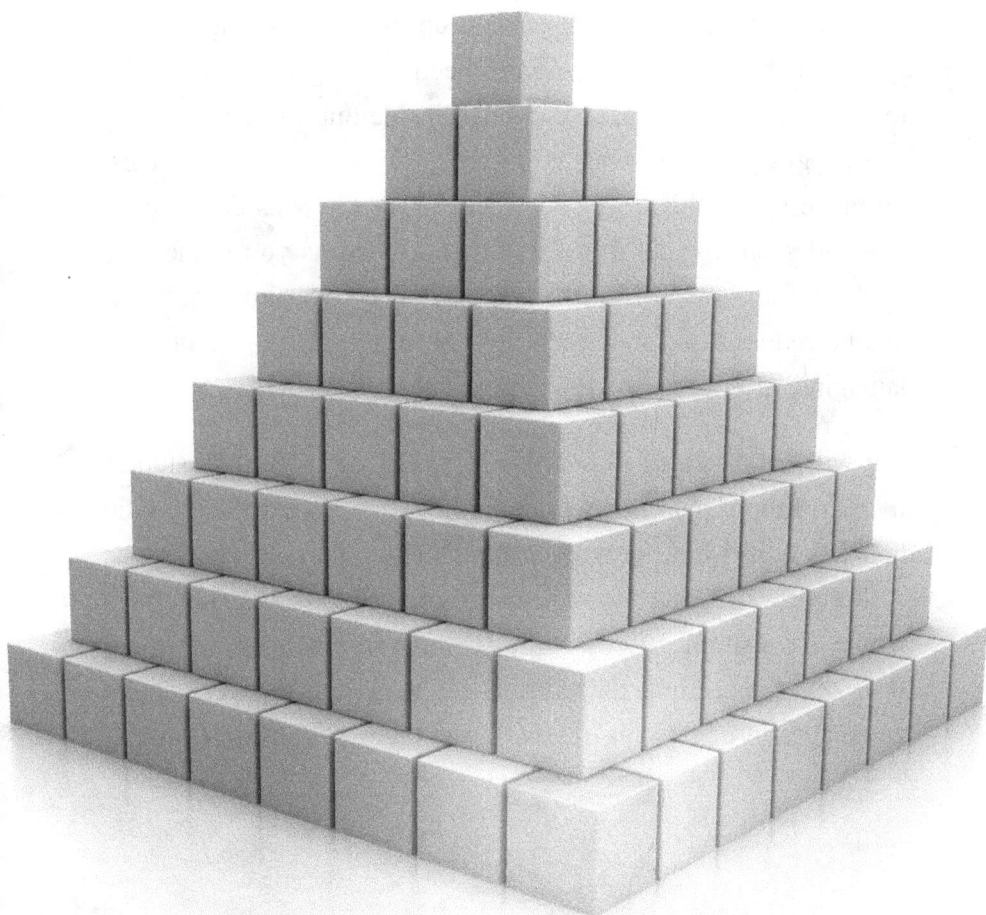

CHAPTER 6

Health's Four Other Cornerstones

1 - The Cholesterol Problem - Or Is It?

So, you have been paying some attention to the prevailing health warnings and advice regarding preventing heart attacks. Understandably so, since the combination of coronary arteries disease, heart attack and strokes add up to being the major cause of deaths in the world. You have been hearing for many years now that the plaques that are created inside our arteries resulting in their gradual narrowing, a process known as atherosclerosis, are made up by this fatty substance we all know as cholesterol. It would seem logical to assume that as long as you reduce the amount of fat in your diet, the cholesterol in your circulation will also be reduced and thus there will be lesser of it to be used as damaging, arterial narrowing material.

You will be surprised to hear however that several large studies involving thousands of individuals have concluded that low-fat diets just don't work, or work long enough to permanently reduce cholesterol. They may lower it for the short term but with most people cholesterol after a while just climbs back up, returning to or often exceeding the original point, so that the real health advantages of dietary fats restrictions are close to insignificant.

> You see, the vast majority of the cholesterol found in
> our arteries is manufactured by our liver,
> in fact some 80%. Only the other 20% actually
> is derived from our food.

Even if you stopped consuming all cholesterol-containing foods, your liver will simply increase its own manufacture, because cholesterol is critical for our life processes, you cannot live without it. A major constituent of our bodies, cholesterol is found in blood, brain tissue, the liver and the kidneys. It forms the walls or membranes of all our cells, our vitamin D and our key regulating hormones, progesterone, estrogen, testosterone and adrenaline.

Of greater importance than the total amount of cholesterol that our bodies manufacture are the mix of the two major types of cholesterol produced. Low-density lipoprotein (LDL) is the 'bad' cholesterol that becomes a threat to our arteries when it undergoes a molecular transformation called oxidisation.

High-density lipoprotein (HDL) is the 'good' cholesterol that transports the bad LDL cholesterol back to the liver for removal out of the bloodstream. For someone with heart concerns, a high level of HDL is one of the best readings to have. The higher the ratio of HDL to LDL, the better protected against developing fatty plaques in your arteries and thus avoiding heart disease you become. Your blood test results will indicate that your good cholesterol should ideally be one quarter of your total cholesterol If your total cholesterol is, for ease of calculation, say 6, than your good cholesterol to prevent plaque formation should ideally be a quarter of that i.e. a HDL level of 1.5. Even better if, and this is a figure that most of our patients will regularly achieve, the ratio is one-third, meaning a higher good cholesterol, HDL level of 2 out of a total cholesterol of 6.

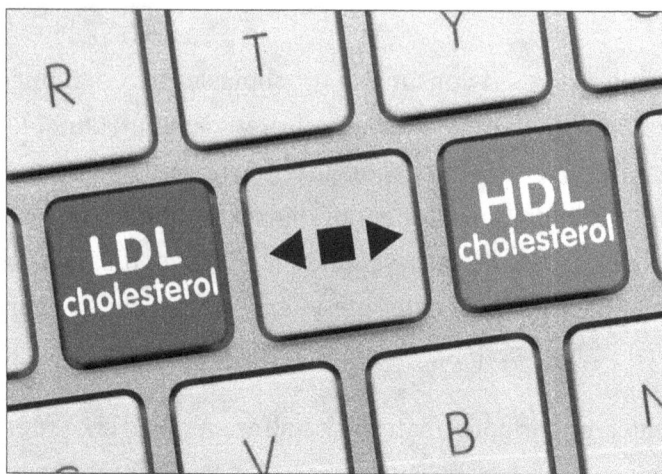

World leading Mayo Clinic has stated and many doctors now agree that your HDL ratio is a more important indicator for predicting the risk of heart disease than your total cholesterol.

They recommend an optimal ratio of 3.5 meaning that with a total cholesterol of 6 ideally the HDL or good cholesterol should be 1.7. Essentially the higher the ratio (i.e. a quarter (HDL of 1.5), a fifth (HDL of 1.2) or a sixth (HDL of 1) etc., the higher the risk of heart disease.

So what is wrong with a low-fat diet? For many, a low-fat diet will often mean feeling hungry again, often shortly after a meal. This will probably cause them to consume greater overall amounts of carbohydrates. These, refined carbohydrates in particular, are, as we have discussed, capable of elevating our blood sugar levels too rapidly causing our pancreas to produce high levels of insulin. High levels of insulin promote the formation of damaging LDL cholesterol as well as causing weight gain and increasing levels of fatigue and tiredness.

> The low-fat and low-cholesterol diets – and therefore by default high carbohydrates – aggressively promoted in the 70s and 80s are largely responsible for the metabolic syndromes, including diabetes and cardiovascular disease which afflict the world today.

Eating a healthier and more satisfying diet, avoiding refined carbohydrates and various stimulants and supplementing their diets with the right natural supplements to help improve the liver functions and reduce oxidisation has assisted many patients at our clinics improve their overall health.

It has also helped improve their physical and mental energy, overall wellbeing and reduce their bad cholesterol (LDL) while increasing their good cholesterol (HDL), therefore improving their cholesterol profiles and reducing their risk of cardiovascular problems dramatically.

2 - Triglycerides

Another very important blood test reading appearing together with your cholesterol results, whose importance is not emphasised nearly enough, sometimes until its levels have gone truly through the roof, are your triglycerides.

Science is not completely clear or how or why, but high triglycerides are frequently associated with not only poorly managed adult onset diabetes and pre-diabetes, but also form part of the group of metabolic disorders which we have been calling hypoglycaemia or metabolic syndrome. Elevated levels of triglycerides are also known to be a side effect of taking some commonly prescribed medications such beta blockers, diuretics, steroids and the birth control pill.

Studies show that it is very common for people with high triglycerides to have low levels of good cholesterol (HDL) and high levels of bad cholesterol (LDL) whilst also suffering with abnormal insulin levels. Therefore, science associates high blood triglycerides levels with a greater risk of the build-up of fatty deposits in the arteries, and is thus regarded as independent risk factors for cardiovascular disease.

> A recent study at Copenhagen Hospital University in Denmark concluded that high triglycerides represent a greater risk of stroke than high levels of cholesterol.

Combined high levels of triglycerides and the bad cholesterol (LDL) increase even more the risk of heart attacks and also some forms of cancer. The Australian Bureau of Statistics indicate that people with high levels of triglycerides had a 54.2% chance of having high levels of total cholesterol, 37.6% chance of higher levels the bad LDL cholesterol, 45.2% more likely to have low levels of good HDL cholesterol, twice as likely to have high blood pressure, and were three times more likely to be diabetic than those with normal levels.

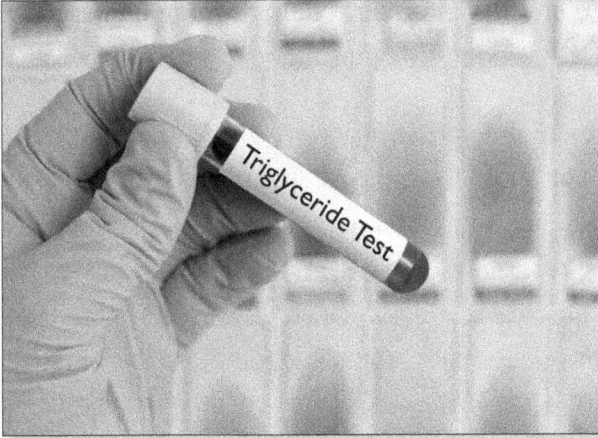

Let us discuss a little more what these triglycerides are and what they do.

Our liver transforms the excessive sugars ingested during our meals or snacking, which the body's cells do not require right now, into glycogen which is stored for later use by the liver as well as by our skeletal muscle.

However the liver and the muscle can only store a limited amount of glycogen and if there are more calories remaining from our meal than there is storage space available in the liver and the muscles, the glucose is transformed into triglycerides and with the help of insulin, stored away, mostly as fatty tissues in our bodies, often in places where we perhaps at times would rather not have them. You may think of triglycerides as efficient batteries, tucked away in our internal organs, hips, buttocks and bellies, for emergency use should the electricity ever get cut off for whatever reason.

So, if one consumes too many calories which the body cannot utilise, particularly easy calories such as carbohydrates and fats, as well as putting on unwanted fat, one could develop higher than desirable levels of triglycerides in one's blood, hypertriglyceridemia.

When we are not eating, in between meals or worse at times of starvation or famine, our blood-sugar levels, as well as our insulin levels, drop and our blood adrenaline rises. The net effect of this causes the release of a fat dissolving enzyme, lipase, which starts the task of breaking down the triglycerides stored in our fatty tissues for release back in our blood where they first came from, to be utilised again as energy.

Triglycerides are substances that can perhaps be easily remembered as a chemical formula resembling the letter "E" in uppercase. The spine of the E shape resembling triglyceride consists of a glycerol molecule and the free legs are each a fatty acid.

Lipase breaks down the stored triglycerides in an orderly and progressive fashion 'one leg' (fatty acid) at the time, transforming it at first to look more like a letter F (or a diglyceride) and then a monoglyceride (kind of a number 7) and then finally a free glycerol spine, without any legs.

By virtue of this formation and breakdown of triglycerides process, twice as much energy can be supplied to our bodies than the energy that could have been directly by sugar alone.

The sugar stored in our muscles in the form of glycogen is reserved for usage by our muscles alone and, in times of fasting or starvation it will not be released or shared with any other organs in our body which are also, at the same time, starving for glucose, such as our brain. However, sugar stored in our liver also in the form of glycogen and which gets changed back into glucose when our blood glucose is low, can and will be released into our blood and shared for use as energy by any organs that require it.

> The sugar storage capacity in our muscles and liver
> is rather limited and can be depleted in a single day.
> The energy stored in the form of triglycerides in our
> fat cells can provide us with energy for up to a
> whole month or more.

The three fatty acids that were being progressively released into our blood during the breakdown of our triglycerides, get absorbed from the blood into our body's cells where they get further broken down for energy utilisation through a process called beta-oxidation. Some of these three fatty acids will also find their way to the liver, where they will also undergo further breaking down into energy generating by-products which include substances known as ketones. The brain, which as mentioned earlier is the major user of the glucose in our blood, can utilise these ketones in lieu of glucose. The remaining (legless) glycerol spine also finds its way into the liver for further breakdown into glucose.

Most blood tests will indicate that normal levels of triglycerides should be somewhere between 0.5 to 1.7 mmol/L in Australia (or 150 mg/dL in the US and some other countries) with 1.7 to 2.2 mmol/L being borderline high and above that either high or very high. It is not unusual for patients to come and see me for their first time at the clinic with recent doctor's blood results on hand showing triglyceride levels of 4, 5 or sometimes even 6, who have not even been warned of their risks. To me even a level of 1.7 mmol/L is not ideal and, soon after our patients begin their treatment program, I aim for and usually get them down, in their next blood test, to at least one half of the 1.7 that is still considered normal. Ideal levels of 0.5 to 0.7 are quite commonly achieved by most of our patients. Contrary to the commonly long held medical belief, we achieve this not by going on an extremely low fat diet, which seldom works anyway, but by simply reducing the excessive carbohydrates, particularly junk food, and implementing a regular protein and good fats dietary program together with the appropriate natural supplements required to improve the liver, the cellular absorption of glucose and its inside of the cell processing into energy.

For these patients their cholesterol levels also improve with results commonly showing a higher levels of good HDL cholesterol and lower bad LDL cholesterol and therefore better HDL to total cholesterol ratios, commonly below 4 and often close to or below 3. The same process slowly reduces the high blood pressure, high insulin levels, normalises blood-sugar levels in diabetics and pre-diabetics, and patients receive the previously mentioned comments from their doctors "whatever you are doing is working so keep it up".

But stabilizing hypoglycaemia or metabolic syndrome isn't all just about diabetes, blood pressure, cholesterol or cardiovascular disease. As a matter of fact hypoglycaemia/metabolic syndrome can and usually does affect virtually everything that everyone almost always presents themselves for in my or any other health practitioner's clinic, as we will discuss a little later on.

Insulin therefore plays an incredible role of beneficial importance when our diet is devoid of useless food, we lead reasonably active lives, our stress levels are under control and we are happily enjoying whatever life brings us, and it can virtually destroy our health and lead to an earlier demise when we don't.

> **It is not just about insulin, it is always all about insulin.**

3 - Homocysteine

Well, for those who thought that the last few pages on triglycerides were somewhat revealing, wait until you hear about the next problem that, particularly when piggybacking on the ones we have just discussed, can increase even more the chance of meeting the world's biggest killers, cardiovascular disease, heart attack and stroke.

The problem is a substance in our blood called homocysteine. Most doctors know about it but many still avoid having their patients levels checked out at blood tests, sometimes even when their cholesterol, triglycerides, blood sugar and blood pressure readings are high, and clearly place the patient in a higher heart attack risk category. It is produced in a biochemical reaction that every cell in our body has to perform in order to be healthy, perform its tasks and survive. This reaction is called methylation.

Don't worry if you don't know much about methylation, most health professionals have only just began hearing about it too. It is a complex reaction but you do not need to know all about it. Few really do and most who claim they do only think so. You only need to know enough to know how high levels of homocysteine affect our bodies and how, if you suspect you could be affected, to get your doctor help you verify it and treat it.

Firstly, how do we get to develop high blood levels of homocysteine (hyperhomocyteinemia) and what problems can it cause?.

Homocysteine is a form of amino acid, that, unlike many of the metabolic problems discussed this far, is not usually brought into our bodies by what we ingest but it could be generated by what we fail to ingest, namely vitamins B6, B12 and folic acid. It could also be caused by genetic problems, which we will also discuss soon.

Higher than normal levels of homocysteine flowing through our arteries have been associated with atherosclerosis and thrombosis which may eventually narrow or block the arteries substantially, reducing the flow of blood and increasing the risk of heart attacks and strokes. Scientists have also noted a strong relationship between high levels of homocysteine in the blood and the narrowing of the carotid artery which brings needed blood to our brains and the presence of which increases another health problem which is also quickly moving towards epidemic proportions – Alzheimer's disease and other types of dementia. Other risks include deep vein thrombosis (DVT) and the lodgement of thrombi into our lungs and thus pulmonary embolism, all serious and life threatening conditions.

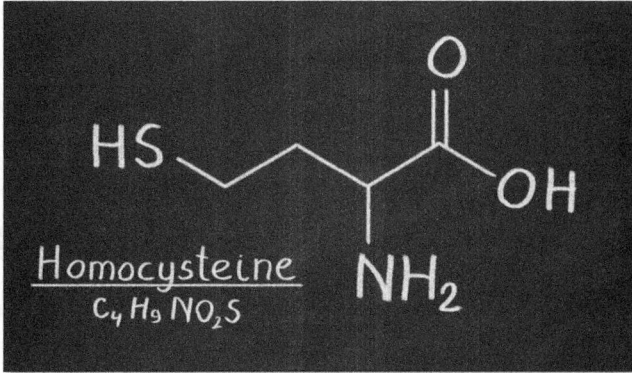

HS

O

OH

Homocysteine
$C_4 H_9 NO_2 S$

NH_2

Other more recent studies have found an association between high levels of blood homocysteine and shortened telomeres in the chromosomes of certain cells particularly leukocytes. Chromosomes are DNA molecules, the programs in the nucleus of the cell that carry all of our genetic information within each one of the trillions of cells that make who we are.

In order for us to be alive, cells need to reproduce and they do so by replication, one mother cell divides into two identical daughter cells. During the replication process each of the strands of chromosomes also duplicate, and are taken into each of the daughter cells with hopefully, the least amount of damage, so that the two photocopies are as close to the original photocopy as possible.

Telomeres are parts of our chromosomes, their tips to be more precise and they play a vital function to protect the chromosome from damage and fusion with other chromosomes when replicating. Telomeres, in their role of protecting the chromosomes, do become damaged and despite there being a regeneration of telomeres process within our bodies, telomeres shortening dysfunction is now recognised as an increased degenerative risk.

Recent studies have found strong evidence that the shortening of telomeres can be strongly influenced by our diets as well as by individual vitamins, particularly folic acid. Therefore, the shortage of folic acid or folate in our bodies is not only one of the possible factors responsible for greater level of homocysteine circulating in our blood and damaging our arteries but also with the faster degeneration of the telomeres placing our chromosomes at greater risk of damage during their replication.

The risks associated with damaged or shortened chromosomal telomeres have been widely investigated by science and include faster cellular aging, risk of cancer, Alzheimer's and Parkinson diseases, rheumatoid arthritis, cardiovascular disease and more. An easier way to explain it is simply to say that the same process that causes high blood levels of homocysteine have been shown in many studies to also damage your telomeres and thus accelerates the ageing process and shortens lives.

Despite the high risk of illness, hospitalisation and mortality associated with high levels of homocysteine, modern medicine is still not recommending to check the blood levels of homocysteine in patients who "have a good diet with plenty of the B group vitamins in it", unless the patient has actually already suffered a heart attack, stroke or a blood clot, or they have a family history of that disease. Unfortunately, many times this will have been too late.

> Finding out after the heart attack or stroke that a simple blood test may have helped you prevent it is unlikely to bring much consolation.

Firstly, even the few people who are very particular about the quality of the food they ingest do not really know today how many vitamins and which vitamins are remaining in the commonly available foods which have been grown in soils depleted of minerals and vitamins, collected, stored transported processed and cooked in ways that almost always reduces the contents of health giving vitamins to at times extremely low and useless amounts.

Secondly, with the prevalence of low hydrochloric acid in many people's stomachs as discussed in our earlier chapters, there is a strong risk of a further reduction in the absorption of what little vitamins are contained in our food. Particularly at risk is vitamin B12 due to intrinsic factor, also already discussed, even if on paper our diet appears to be good, do we really know what we are absorbing and what we are not?

Thirdly, how often and when was the last time that your doctor thoroughly, or even not so thoroughly, questioned and discussed your diet to be able to determine whether you are likely to be absorbing and utilising your essential nutrients including vitamins B6, B12 and folate required to neutralise homocysteine and prevent the corresponding risks?

If he or she did, as I hope they will have, then they are probably a good, well informed doctor, and fortunately these days there are more and more around who dare to think outside the square and you should definitely stick with them.

The reason for their reluctance is because all medical and scientific observations of the effects of high blood homocysteine with coronary artery disease (CAD), heart attacks and strokes have not as yet been proven with absolute certainty, even though science accepts that high homocysteine is present in twice the number of people who suffer with these conditions than those who do not.

I guess tobacco companies also insisted for many prolonged years that because it could not be proven beyond the shadow of a doubt that smoking caused cancer even though smokers had a much higher rate of cancer than non-smokers, that therefore smoking was safe.

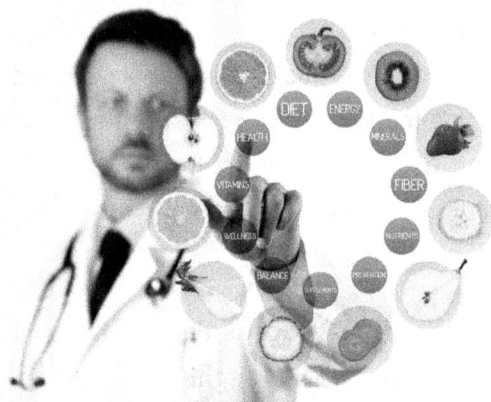

Whilst some may argue that the analogy may not completely apply to homocysteine, do you really want to wait for a few decades before science has more than just the current anecdotal evidence that the high homocysteine levels present in most cardiovascular disease victims is one of the major reasons for their condition?

I am sure that the smokers who had the vision of quitting smoking, even without seeing the smoking gun that proved that nicotine caused lung cancer, were very happy to have made the early choice of having done so. Particularly when the treatment for reducing high homocysteine problem does not have to be anywhere as challenging as giving up sugars or cigarettes.

4 – MTHFR

Let's find about a little more how homocysteine is formed in our bodies.

Homocysteine is a naturally occurring amino formed in our bodies during a very important cellular biochemical reaction called methylation.

As stated earlier, the complete biochemistry of methylation can be very complex and I will therefore try to keep it within the practical context of this book by simplifying it and skipping large chunks of the full purpose and biochemistry of methylation.

To start with, let's attempt to define methylation. Methylation is yet another very important function which occurs behind the scenes in our bodies and if it all goes well, we just take it for granted. After all who wants to spend time asking our bodies if they have methylated well today, nor congratulate our methylation process for contributing to us having had an enjoyable day full of vitality. However, we may certainly become very aware of its effects on our health and wellbeing should this process ever get out of balance.

The purpose of the methylation process is to add or more correctly transfer a molecule called a 'methyl group' to another substance, such as, for example, our DNA or a protein, so that the DNA or the protein receiving this methyl group may be able to perform whatever functions they are meant to perform.

As you can imagine both the DNA and proteins are the basis and the building blocks of life and are involved in a myriad of functions. Without methylation transferring the methyl group molecule in say our bone cells, they will develop problems in performing their function which is to produce healthy bone, hair cells for hair to grow, brain cells to perform a large number of different brain functions, etc., etc. It is during this methylation process that homocysteine, as well as other important molecules, is produced.

Probably the easiest way to visualise the methylation process is to think of a wall clock whose hour hands are going around and around.

The diagram below is a very simplified version of the methylation process to make it easier to explain the basic concept. For the readers who may become fascinated by this process and wish to get a more in-depth understanding, there is no shortage of information on the net together with far more detailed biochemical diagrams where the complexity is such as to make all the lines look like a bowl of spaghetti.

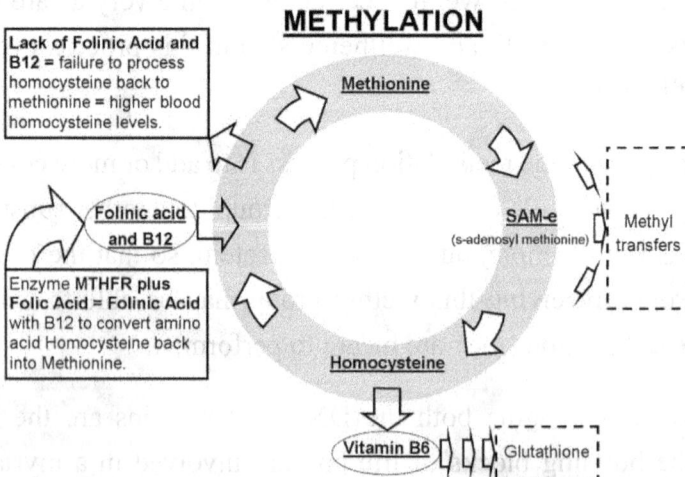

METHYLATION

Lack of Folinic Acid and B12 = failure to process homocysteine back to methionine = higher blood homocysteine levels.

Methionine

Folinic acid and B12

Enzyme MTHFR plus Folic Acid = Folinic Acid with B12 to convert amino acid Homocysteine back into Methionine.

SAM-e (s-adenosyl methionine)

Methyl transfers

Homocysteine

Vitamin B6

Glutathione

The methylation process begins at the 12 o'clock position on the above diagram, with an essential amino acid called methionine. Essential because the body is not capable of making its own methionine and should it not be in your food, then you will become short of it, with dire consequences for your health because of the many roles it plays. The best source of methionine are eggs, sesame seeds, cheese and brazil nuts but is also abundant in fish, meat and poultry.

Through a series of chemical reactions occurring between the 12 o'clock and 3 o'clock segments, methionine changes to s-adenisyl-methionine (SAM-e) at the 3 o'clock position in the diagram. The production of SAM-e is really the most important part of this cycle because it is SAM-e that donates or transfers the methyl group to the DNA, protein etc.

SAM-e then proceeds with a number of different reactions and changes and resurfaces at the 6 o'clock position on the diagram in the form of homocysteine.

Homocysteine, as you will have gathered by now, is really not desirable in our bodies in high quantities because of it being associated with a number of life risking and shortened biochemical activities. However, homocysteine is still essential, just not in high amounts, because driven by vitamin B6 it is capable of undergoing a series of changes which culminate through a process called transsulfuration with the production of glutathione, probably the most important and powerful antioxidant in our bodies. If homocysteine is too low, there may then not be enough of it to convert back to methionine at 12 o'clock and this could bring the cycle to a grinding halt.

So, homocysteine needs to undergo further reactions mainly driven by folinic acid, which is the activated form of folic acid, and vitamin B12 to transform it back to methionine, where it all started at the 12 o'clock position. The same cycle will then recommence, over and over again to keep on producing SAM-e for the purpose to keep transferring the methyl group.

The most common problem in this cycle is the lack of vitamins B6, B12 and folinic acid in the diet, causing a failure to break down homocysteine at the 9 o'clock position and change it back to methionine. When this occurs, homocysteine blood levels raise and associate themselves with the various health problems already discussed.

Some health care professionals had been aware for several decades that any patients coming to see them with high cholesterol, diabetes or cardiovascular problems and also high homocysteine required the lowering of this amino acid to lessen the patient's risk of greater health problems.

I remember decades ago regularly telling my patients with high homocysteine that they had a very good chance of reducing it by supplementing with vitamins B6, B12 and folic acid, the most commonly available supplement form of the folinic acid. It would almost always work and work very well, but not always and occasionally, for reasons which only became obvious many years later, we could not reduce the homocysteine at all.

Well, one of the reasons for some people failing to reduce their homocysteine has become obvious to science in just the last few years and not too many health practitioners understand it nor believe in it as yet.

You see, methylation requires 'folinic acid'. Most supplements contain 'folic acid'. The names are almost identical but folic acid cannot play the role of folinic acid which is required at the 9 o'clock position in our diagram. However, we knew from our nutritional biochemistry education that we all had an enzyme in our bodies which could change folic acid to folinic acid. The enzyme has a long name of **methylenetetrahydrofolate reductase** or MTHFR for short.

> It is only a relatively recent discovery that not everyone's MTHFR enzymes are capable of changing folic acid into folinic acid, because of genetic errors.

These days many blood testing laboratories can do a blood test that lets you know the most common genetic defects that may render the gene in charge of encoding or causing the production of the MTHFR enzyme to be defective. Although there are more than 40 known MTHFR defects, there are two genes on our number one chromosome, one in position 677 and the other in position 1298 which have been studied the most and at the moment seem to carry the greatest health consequences. Unfortunately not many health professionals have even looked at this test for their patients as yet.

The genetic defects may affect the nucleotide encoding positions 677 only, 1298 only, or both. The defect may have been inherited from one parent only (heterozygous) or both (homozygous). If the blood test shows that there are no defects in either position, then we should be able to change folic acid into folinic acid without any real problems and allow homocysteine to break down into methionine.

If we only have a defect on say position 677 from one parent (heterozygous) our ability to change folic acid into folinic is estimated to be reduced by 40%, if homozygous then 70%. If 1298 is heterozygous there is a 20% loss of function and if homozygous a 40% loss. If both 677 and 1298 are heterozygous, then the term used is compound heterozygous with a 50% loss of function.

MTHFR Gene Mutations

Gene	Hetero-zygous Loss of function	Homo-zygous Loss of function	Combined Hetero-zygous Loss of function
C677T	40%	70%	50%
A1298C	20%	40%	

So far we have only discussed how genetic defects with our MTHFR enzyme can cause high levels of homocysteine in our blood. Unfortunately defective MTHFR enzymes can cause other repercussions within the methylation process, because if homocysteine does not change into methionine and the methionine levels from our diet also happen to be low because of other health stresses that confiscate even more of this already lacking amino acid, the SAM-e levels can also drop. SAM-e at 3 o'clock on the diagram is where the accomplishment of good methylation, the production of methyl groups, gets passed on to the many functions in the body which require this methyl group.

Case Study no. 17 – Pam's personal testimonial.

I met Bruno many years ago when suffering with extremely unstable blood-sugar levels. The levels read from extremely high to alarmingly and dangerously low. My GP was unable to help me, so on recommendation I contacted Bruno Marevich. He put me on a regime that brought me back from the brink of diabetes. His knowledge was far superior to others that I had spoken to and I am so very grateful for his help.

Some months ago I, unfortunately contracted a nasty virus and eventually became 'chronically fatigued'. I contacted Bruno and was overjoyed to find that I could see him soon for an appointment. Again, with his vast knowledge, encouragement and medication, I have gone from being bedridden to leading a normal life.

Bruno Marevich is THE most knowledgeable and genuinely conscientious man (health provider/naturopath) I have ever known. I would turn to him before anyone else and have recommended him to many, many people.

Pam S.

> **COMMENTS:** There was a time when Pam was so fatigued she could hardly get out of bed. We treated her digestive tract and blood-sugar metabolism and since then her health and energy have improved considerably. However, even though Pam is quite positive about her great improvements, she is still prone to episodes of fatigue and tiredness. In the last few years, with more laboratories beginning to test for MTHFR, I have asked Pam to have a blood test, which found Pam positive for compound heterozygous, a 50% loss of MTHFR function, casting more light on the reasons for her inability of living a completely fatigue free life up to now. As well as using activated B group vitamins these days we are also working at harmonising the many other biochemical reactions involved in methylation. Pam's spirit is very determined to keep on working to get this unasked-for condition under control and is diligently following our current test trials to help us become more aware of her specific treatment and supplementation requirements.

Also, folinic acid on its own, is not only required for methylation in the body but also serves many other important functions. The consequences of low SAM-e and low folinic acid can therefore amount to even more problems and more symptoms to challenge your health care provider, including depression, anxiety, tiredness, poor sleep patterns, poor red and white blood cell production, the "on and off" switching of inflammatory reactions, more rapid cellular ageing, poor detoxification of chemicals, impaired energy production, greater risk of neural tube disorders and spina bifida. People with this condition may also often develop eye problems, abnormal blood clotting, skeletal abnormalities, allergies, schizophrenia and other cognitive problems.

Wow, what a long list, but to complicate matters even further if possible the cells of untreated MTHFR defects sufferers will often not be able to deal properly with natural medication either such as herbs, minerals and vitamins. This makes them further prone to poor health and disease and presents the practitioner with many challenges requiring particular knowledge and experience of this condition in order to help the patient.

From a methylation cycle and a vitamins standpoint therefore you will be quite rightly beginning to suspect that the B complex group of vitamins plays a vital role in keeping this important process working particularly, B6 and B12. And, for not only those people with a genetic loss of function of their MTHFR enzyme but for everyone else too, also the activated form of folic acid i.e. folinic acid.

However, I hope that I have by now been able to also get some of the message across that our bodies are not simply an aggregate of many complex biochemical reactions, all of which can be fixed by just dropping-in the required drugs or missing biochemical ingredients where they are needed. Indeed this form of healing is very often the standard approach applied by many modern-day health care professionals.

Whilst not denying in any way that supplementing with specific vitamins and at times perhaps also drugs that target the specific problem or malfunction will often bring a level of relief and perhaps also some repair, true health and healing should be a process that enlists the cooperative assistance of the whole body, as well as our minds, and in particular our digestive tracts and blood glucose metabolism.

These two alone do not constitute our whole body but they are, in my opinion and in those of the tens of thousands of people I have helped at my clinics, the two main problems that this day and age are more likely to stop our bodies from being healthy.

> Fix correctly your digestive tract and improve your sugar metabolism and your body will not fail to get itself back into a 'healing mode'.

This will either take care of your health problems or will at least improve the chances that whatever other work your body may require, whether they be medicines or supplements for the specific problem that is worrying you, will have a greater chance to work well for you. A healthy body takes care of all of its problems better than one which is not.

CHAPTER 7

The Marevich Way (TMW) to Energy and Health

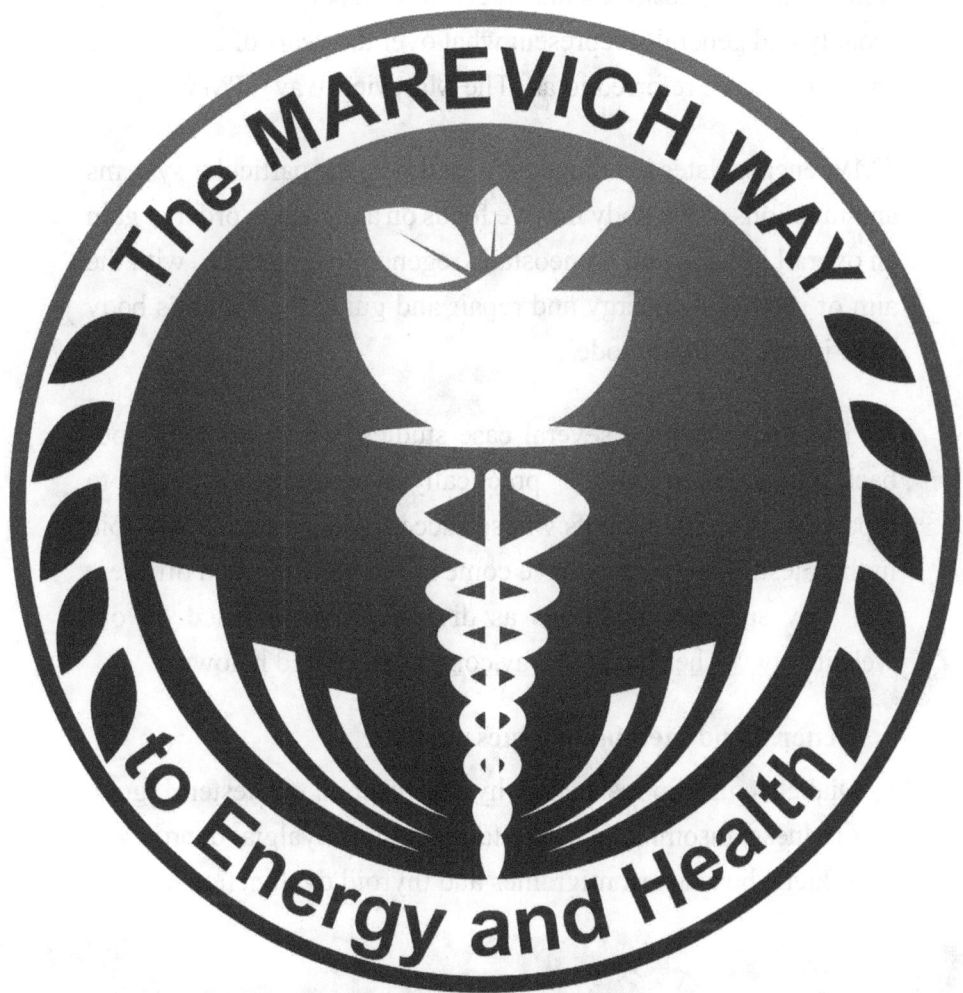

CHAPTER 7

The Marevich Way (TMW) to Energy and Health

The naturopathic and scientific methods of treatment outlined and discussed in some detail so far in this book, accompanied by case studies based on testimonials received from some of our patients, broadly and generally represent what over the years of clinical use has grown to be referred to as 'The Marevich Way' (TMW).

TMW encapsulates the diagnostic methods, the particular systems and functions of the body that we focus on and treat in order to gain an overall holistic and homeostatic regenerative reaction, with the aim of promoting energy and repair and guide the patient's body back into a 'healing mode'.

As it's clear from the several case studies, when the body goes back into a "healing mode" practically everything else begins to repair. Most of the patients whose success stories are happily told in their testimonials, may have come to see us with often different and very specific conditions as diverse as those listed on our website www.TheMarevichWay.com.au and listed below:

- **General and metabolic issues such as:**

  Diabetes, insulin resistance, hypoglycaemia, cholesterol, gout, tiredness, insomnia, chronic fatigue, fibromyalgia, depression, anxiety, headaches, migraines and thyroid dysfunctions.

- **Digestive tract problems including:**

  Reflux, constipation, irritable bowel, ulcerative colitis, Crohn's, celiac and helicobacter pylori.

- **Immune system related condition:**

  Respiratory problems such as colds, asthma sinusitis as well as skin conditions such as psoriasis, eczema, acne and dermatitis plus other allergies, intolerances and sensitivities and autoimmune disorders.

- **Hormonal and fertility difficulties including:**

  Period problems, menopausal issues, endometriosis, fibroids, polycystic ovaries, female and male fertility.

- **Cardiovascular issues including:**

  Heart problems, cardiomyopathies, atherosclerosis, circulation problems and blood pressure

- **Muscular and skeletal conditions including:**

  Lower back and sciatica problems, neck and shoulder pain including headaches and migraines and we specialise in the Myorthotics treatment technique.

Despite the length of this list, it covers only the most common conditions we help patients using TMW day in and day out. The practical success of TMW has been constant and predictable. The exceptionally vast percentage of the tens of thousands of patients we have helped, have all been assisted using the standard TMW program. The same can thus be also said for all the short testimonials at the front of the book as well as for all the listed case studies scattered throughout it.

Some patients, perhaps 10% overall, have had to have the standard TMW program tweaked and adjusted to fit their particular condition or sensitivity (i.e. children, pregnant and lactating mothers, patients with unusual food sensitivities or genetic defects, patients requiring extra symptomatic support whilst the real causes of their condition were being treated, such as chronic arthritis sufferers, patients suffering with heavy depression or anxiety, etc.). The changes from the standard TMW for these people would normally be in the form of some dietary changes from our standard hypoglycaemic diet or an increase or reduction of supplements.

Again, the vast majority of our patients, regardless of their specific, medically diagnosed or not condition, will start and finish their treatment on the standard TMW program.

TMW

Now, let's get down to nitty gritty and discuss the process that most patients coming to our clinic go through.

To summarise TMW, these are its main components:

1. Take the patient's health history and medical reports if any.

2. Carry out eye diagnosis to define the patients constitutional condition and any significant signs relating to their present health.

3. Explain the findings to the patient and the proposed treatment and how this is expected to assist in the improvement of the specific condition/s they have come to see us for.

4. Explain hypoglycaemic diet.

5. Explain supplements, why they are being prescribed and how they are to be taken.

6. Explain any possible detox symptoms that occasionally manifest themselves in the first few days of the treatment. We request that they call the clinic to discuss any detox effects or any concerns should they arise. Indeed in our clinic all our new patients are entitled to free telephone support during their first month to make them feel secure that if they need us they should have no reasons not to call us.

7. We ask the patient to come back in two weeks' time for their first follow-up visit. At that stage they usually feel better, they have questions, we have questions. We ensure that they are following and understanding TMW program to the best of their abilities. At this stage most patients are seeing improvement and are pleased and excited about what is going on. Occasionally same may take a little longer.

8. Patients then come back in two more weeks to ensure all is proceeding well. By now most patients are well out of detox, have better energy all day long, tend to sleep more deeply all night long and get up in the morning feeling refreshed and finding it easier to get out of bed.

9. At that stage, even though most patients feel already much better than in some cases they had felt for years, it is kind-of all done with mirrors. It takes normally longer for most patients to have had sufficient repair in their gastrointestinal tract and resensitisation of their cellular membranes to allow better response to insulin signalling by the glucose receptors.

10. From here on, where required, we will continue to see the patient a few more times , usually on a four-weekly basis to ensure they remain feeling on top of the wave as they continue with their endeavour to repair as much as their bodies will allow this program to repair. Most patients have by now become quite used to feeling good and are committed to TMW. Some will make mistakes or take occasional departures from time to time, with food choices mainly, but will soon return to their proper path. Everyone tries the best they can and everyone enjoys the benefits derived from TMW.

11. When a certain stability has been reached and their bodies are capable of handling things on their own, some patients conclude the program and return to see us from time to time should anything change. Many will feel better than they have ever done and will want to continue taking a reduced maintenance dosage of the required supplements and try to follow the philosophy of the diet, which they are now used to, as much as they can. Some will go back to a few of the old dietary habits i.e. the odd cup of coffee, glass of wine or a sweet, but the progress that they have made and the continued support from some of the supplements will generally see them in very good condition for the rest of their lives, which will already have been statistically prolonged because of having enrolled in TMW program.

12. When we see them again from time to time they will continue to report that they have never again been bothered by whatever brought them to see us in the first place, be they migraines, ulcers, cholesterol, tiredness, etc., etc. and will happily report

that they hardly get any colds, if they do they are only mild and quick to pass.

> Most importantly, their lives will almost always have changed for the better. The newly found energy gave them the confidence to move on in life and tackle opportunities that they may just not have been confident enough with their past energy and health condition to take on.

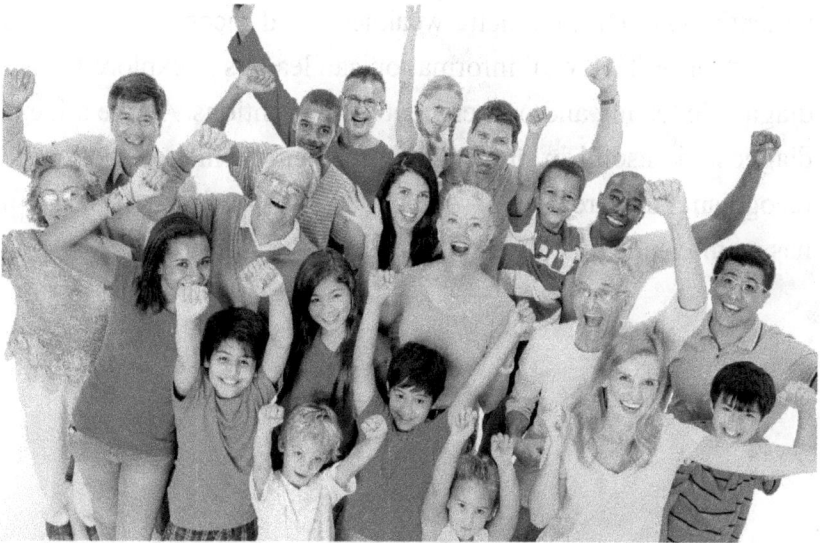

Eye Diagnosis

Apart from taking health history and examining other available medical tests, we will also, using a specialised microscope, carry out an 'eye diagnosis' of each patient to help us identify issues about their bodies which are useful to a naturopath.

For those who do not know, this is not actually an eye test to determine the physical condition of the eyes.

Eye diagnosis gives us the tools to see disease potential in the patient's body (from genetic weakness) and recognise metabolic individuality. This vital information can lead us to explore further diagnostic testing and/or therapeutic interventions. Above all, eye diagnosis is useful in preventative medicine which is the key to recognising and treating an organ weakness or function before it has manifested clinically as a disease.

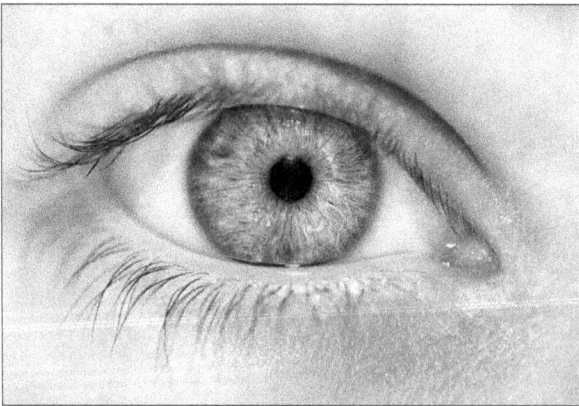

Most of what is known today about eye diagnosis has come to us from Germany, where this form of diagnosis has a very strong and reputable basis. Many medical practitioners in Germany are reputed to be using eye diagnosis as part of their diagnostic armoury.

The term 'eye diagnosis' refers more accurately than 'iris diagnosis' or the more commonly used term 'iridology' which refers specifically to the study of the iris. Eye diagnosis employs the study of other parts of the eye as well including the pupil, sclera, conjunctiva and retina. Therefore eye diagnosis is also, even more correctly, called the study of 'ophthalmological phenomena'.

A good eye diagnostician, like any other health professional must start with the assumption that each patient is an individual. Each person is unique. This means that any system of diagnosis, including eye diagnosis, should not be looked as an exact science but also an art.

In practiced hands, eye diagnosis is an extremely valuable tool because the signs in the eye indicate most aspects of a person's state of health.

Despite many theories as to how the inherited conditions and predispositions in our bodies, as well as the changes that have taken place during the degradation of our health or for that matter during its improvement, are exactly transposed through to the eyes, is still subject to research. Most theories are essentially based on the fact that the nerves that link our brain to every part of our body as well as the myriads of chemical reactions occurring non-stop in every one of our cells, and a lot of this massive amount of information is reported back to our brain.

The eyes are simply an extension to the brain and just as the massive amounts of information from our environment get captured by our eyes and get transferred to the brain, information from inside us gets transmitted to the brain which reflects it in our eyes.

Indeed the eye's retina and optic nerve are a part of the brain, as during early development a small part of the brain pouches out and becomes the retina and optic nerve. The eye is therefore the only part of our brain which can be seen directly – it happens when the optician shines a bright light and looks at the retina, the innermost layer of our eye and the optic nerve that carries visual information to the brain, the most complex arrangement of matter in the known universe.

"The eyes are the windows to our body." Although this is an explanation lacking any scientific depth for the moment and does not fully explain what happens in currently known or understood scientific terms, with the advent of quantum mechanics and epigenetics, new frontiers of knowledge are becoming exposed and available for the greater understanding of the role the eyes play as a diagnostic tool to make us more aware of our body's health.

The Nutritional Program

As explained in detail in Chapter 4, there is virtually no one whose blood-sugar regulation is even close to what it should be from the very young to the very old. Most of the populations' blood glucose will have been subjected to trips on a highs and lows roller coaster way before the children even mature to school age.

One may agree to this on the basis of having heard that it is a disease that can be attributed primarily to a greater prosperity in the western world than ever before in history. Whilst there is certainly some truth in this, you may be surprised that Asia and Africa rank just as high and are quickly increasing, with over 100 million diabetics in China alone.

Over the years we have strived to develop a diet that would suit the vast majority of our patients. It had to be nutritionally well balanced, provide sufficient energy but also empower healthy weight loss (as can be seen by the many weight loss reports in this book's testimonials) as well as help improve other health scourges such as diabetes, out of balance cholesterol levels, blood pressure, digestive problems, and to encourage good bacterial growth and a healthy intestine. It had to be able to be used by most people with only small modifications, from the young to the old. Not a lot to ask.

We developed the hypoglycaemic diet by researching, studying and testing out other nutritional plans, some old and others more modern. Guess what, after giving it to several thousand patients and seeing continuous superior results than any other diets when used in conjunction with our supplements, we wondered why we should not give it to each and every one of our patients. With a few notable exceptions – being those patients who have opted for whatever reasons, mostly moral or religious to be vegetarians or vegans – all of our other patients are placed on a hypoglycaemic eating program as part of TMW.

Best decision we ever made, now whole families that come to see us (mum has hormonal problems and would like to lose some weight, dad has high cholesterol and feels tired, daughter feels tired too and has embarrassing skin outbreaks, son gets frequent colds and asthma attacks that cause him to take a lot of time from school and not be able to participate in school or other sports, grandpa has blood pressure and reflux and grandma has bad arthritis and chest pains) are on the same TMW diet.

They can all get rid of the same wrong foods in the house and mum and grandma do not have to cook different meals for everyone in the house.

> Best of all, despite their very different starting conditions, they all get healthier whilst on the same program, feel better and the doctor can then start reducing their medicinal drugs.

The three main rules for the hypoglycaemic diet are:

1. DO NOT LET YOUR BLOOD-SUGAR DROP LOW

    To help stabilise blood-sugar levels, some food should be consumed during the day at regular intervals not greater than three hours apart. It is important to be 'proactive' - don't wait for your blood sugar to drop before having some food. Use a 'stepping-stone' approach: i.e., eat enough at breakfast to last until morning tea and so on knowing that the next meal is not too far away and you need not go hungry.

2. RAISE YOUR BLOOD-SUGAR SLOWLY

    As a general rule, the faster your blood-sugar level goes up, the faster it also falls back down. Therefore, all foods which cause blood sugar to rise too rapidly must be avoided or restricted (mainly simple but also some other starchy carbohydrates).

3. EAT A BALANCED DIET

The ideal balance, to give sufficient cell building food, energy building foods and fibre for the bacteria in the gastrointestinal tract is two-thirds complex carbohydrates (vegetables, fruits, nuts, seeds, grains, wholemeal pastas/breads/flour, brown rice, lentil, etc.) and at least one-third animal protein (fish, poultry, meats and eggs). It is essential that some animal protein be consumed at each major meal (breakfast, lunch and dinner – breakfast being most important).

A full copy of TMW hypoglycaemic diet which these days we give to each and every one of our patients who we also closely instruct, monitor, help modify and tweak if necessary when required, can be downloaded from: **www.TheMarevichWay.com.au**

We thought we would make the diet available on our website rather than in this book, as this allows us to keep it up to date with any refinements or new explanations and you are then sure to be able to obtain its latest version.

It is obvious that all diets should ideally be carried out with the support of a qualified practitioner. It is impossible for any diet, no matter how good, to suit each and every person on this large planet as there will always be an exception.

> Therefore we recommend that you should only start any dietary programme, ours included, after discussing your specific case with a qualified practitioner.

Supplements

I was fortunate enough as explained earlier in the book to have been mentored by extraordinary naturopaths. People would queue up to go see them and would always get the results they were hoping to get and often more than they expected. One thing some of these practitioners had in common in those days was that they knew a lot about which forms and combinations of vitamins worked and which ones did not.

Also, the right good vitamins were not so easy to find so that some naturopaths who had started practicing some thirty or forty years before I ever saw my first patient, were also making their own vitamins. My foremost mentor, Robert Lucy already owned an ultramodern supplements manufacturing plant in Castle Hill which was fully registered with the Australian regulating authorities, staffed with workers, chemists and PhD-level staff focused on producing leading edge, high quality vitamins.

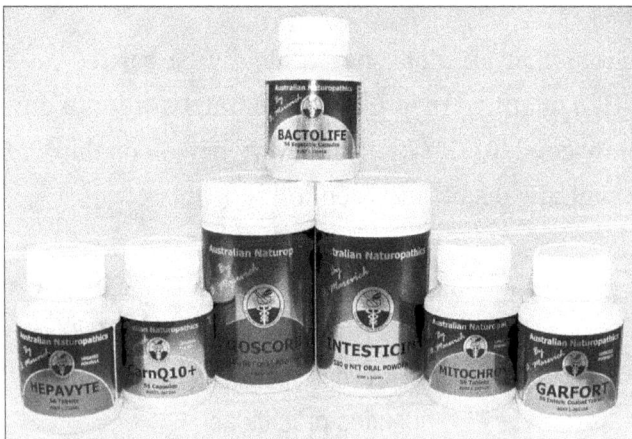

What a better person for me to learn all about formulating, manufacturing and prescribing vitamins than a man who in order to give the right nutrients to the patients who were knocking the doors down to come and see him many years ago had only one choice at that time – to make them himself. Many of the current day better known and well reputed brands found in health food shops and pharmacies also started off in this way.

That start continued my intense love affair with finding the best combination of individual nutrient ingredients that when properly combined together would benefit almost every one and almost every condition.

Most of the supplements we have been prescribing to our patients for the last almost 20 years are the Australian Naturopathics brand of products, all formulated by us and manufactured in Australia under stringent good manufacturing practice (GMP) regulations by large, ultra-modern pharmaceutical products contract manufacturers. We regularly prescribe and supply the following broad categories of supplements to practically every patient, for almost every condition:

A) For the gastrointestinal tract and the liver:

- Supplement 1: Herbs and vitamins which will REMOVE the bad bacteria from the gastrointestinal tract and at the same time also help reduce overall inflammation.

- Supplement 2: Herbs and vitamins which will help REPAIR and regrow the villi and the mucosal lining of the intestine.

- Supplement 3: Prebiotics and probiotics to supply the digestive tract with healthy intestinal bacteria.

- Supplement 4: Herbs and vitamins to facilitate the liver detoxification process, stabilise the liver function and help regenerate and regrow health liver cells, hepatocytes.

B) To reduce damaging oxidative stress:

- Supplement 5: Vitamins and minerals which will act as electron donors i.e. antioxidants and immune system boosters.

C) To improve the absorption of nutrients at cellular level:

- Supplement 6: A formulation consisting mainly of B group vitamins and herbs that allow the biochemical processing of carbohydrates for energy production in our cells.

- Supplement 7: A formulation which assists the absorption and processing of fatty acids by the cells in the body by helping the fatty acids cross the cellular membrane and process these into energy.

These seven groups of vitamins are meant to address the areas and functions that you want to be able to get your vitamins to affect, influence and improve. We have purposely stayed away from nominating the specific name of each vitamin, herb or mineral. There are a very large number of vitamins available these days and they all have varying or sometimes slightly different ingredients used to try to achieve the same result. For example when talking about antioxidants, apart from the well-known vitamin C there are many other vitamins that are better or not as good antioxidants.

The best way to find a formula or brand that suits you and your condition best is to approach someone who deals with vitamins at a chemist shop and ask for a good antioxidant for someone with your condition. The same applies to all the seven group of vitamins mentioned above. You can therefore use this list of groups of supplements when you go to a health food shop, pharmacy or, my recommendation is that you see a naturopath that has been recommended to you by someone who has already had good results from following their advice.

The internet is these days a storehouse of vitamins information. Whenever ordering any vitamins you would be well served to ensure they fit into the category of vitamins that attempt to treat the problem not just the symptoms. Losing hair for example will almost always also be a warning sign of your digestive tract and blood-sugar levels affecting other important functions such as your absorption of essential nutrients, possibly the function of your thyroid, hormonal system, circulation etc. If at all possible do not just get sold a hair strengthening formula. It may well help your hair somewhat but you will just be turning off the warning signs that something could be going wrong in your body.

Author's Final Thoughts

If I could summarise on one page or two all the knowledge that I have learned from my experience and the research of others in the field of medicine, science, thought processes and complementary medicine or natural therapies, I would say as follows:

1. A healthy body can prevent many illnesses and diseases before they even start and if you are unlucky to get struck down with a condition anyway, it will help you get over it sooner. Survival of the fittest. **Preventing is better than curing.**

2. If you become unwell, tired or ill, by all means see your doctor but also try to identify the foods, lifestyle, attitudes and beliefs about yourself and others that may have contributed to your health's deterioration. If you cannot do this on your own, **find an experienced naturopath or complementary medicine practitioner** who can.

3. In your endeavours to recover and become healthier, regardless of the nature of your condition, you will never go wrong if you focus on restoring optimal health to your digestive tract, liver and balance well your blood-sugar. They may not fix you up completely every time but will at least make your other efforts to get better much more likely to work. **Treat the causes, not just the symptoms.**

4. Take time to find out which supplements really work at fixing the core of all problems and not just the symptoms that you are exhibiting and use those daily.

These days vitamins and minerals are no longer in your food. Think of the expense of regularly buying good supplements as an essential part of your family's weekly groceries bill. See it as a great investment into a more advantaged life. They will give you a much better quality of life, almost certainly prolong it whilst enjoying more of all our creator has gifted us.

5. Eat healthy foods, avoid sugars as well as refined and chemically adulterated products. **Medicinal drugs are unlikely to prevent diseases so take them only if you have absolutely no choice.** Be hygienic, minimise your exposure to all radiations, enjoy at least eight hours of good sleep every night, breathe clean air, drink fresh water, let the sun and good fresh air regularly caress your skin, exercise and rest regularly and let the world be a better place for your having been here.

6. **Always be happy**. If at times you are not, your first priority is to go back to a high vibrating level of consciousness where you can sense the resonance of calm, positive expectations, gratefulness and appreciation and a love and deeply burning desire for more and more life resonating right through your heart and bones. Thank your Creator. Whatever you believe in with complete certainty, will not fail to be given to you, including good health

7. **Make Your Health Great Again!**

Bruno Marevich
Naturopath.

About the Author

Bruno Marevich

Author, Naturopath, and Neuro Linguistics Programming Practitioner

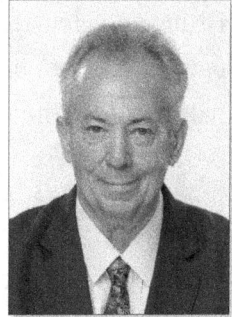

Deeply interested in natural medicine, health and science from an early age, he initially graduated in accounting due to the lack of formal courses in the field of natural medicine at that time in Australia. In the early 1980s, Bruno began his studies in naturopathy. He went on to earn an Advanced Diploma of Naturopathy followed by a university degree in Health Sciences majoring in Complimentary Medicine. He also earned his Master Practitioner qualification in Neuro Linguistic Programming.

Bruno has been helping patients for over three decades, consulting from his clinic in Castle Hill, New South Wales for the past 15 years and before that in his Macquarie Street clinic in Sydney. Happily married to his wife Henriette for 39 years, he credits her keen interest, enthusiasm, tireless support, positive thinking and love for their success over the years.

Their wish, goal, and desire has always been to alleviate pain and suffering while bringing health, energy, and propelling motivation to the lives of all who have sought their advice. He and his wife have been fortunate to have met tens of thousands of patients. Their greatest reward has been the improvement in the life of everyone they meet and those who experience the profound benefits of nature's healing.

Bruno and Henriette founded the Australian Naturopathics brand of natural supplements in the year 2000 for the purpose of providing patients with their own formulas of high quality natural medicinal products. These form today an integral part of their naturopathic treatment which has come to be known as 'The Marevich Way'.

Bruno's professional associations include the Complementary Medicine Association (CMA) for which he was a Director and Federal Secretary for many years. The CMA contributes to Australians who seek help from naturopaths and to the profession by working towards the improvement of naturopathic educational standards and code of practice. This organisation also helped increase the number of private health funds which today covers naturopathy in Australia. He has been awarded a fellowship to the Complementary Medicine Association in recognition for his extensive service to the naturopathic profession. Bruno is also a member of the New York Academy of Sciences and Civil Liberties Australia.

In his spare time, Bruno enjoys a healthy personal fitness routine and he is an avid snow skier. He also passionately continues his personal studies and professional research in the fields of science, medicine, biochemistry, nutrition, psychology and quantum physics. Bruno is in constant search for the truth about health and ways of improving mankind's condition.

He has travelled and worked repeatedly throughout more than 30 countries to date and continues to attend professional health events and conventions across the world, which he manages to squeeze in with his clinic's busy schedule.

Bruno Marevich is the author of *Make Your Health Great Again* and lives in Sydney NSW, with his wife Henriette.

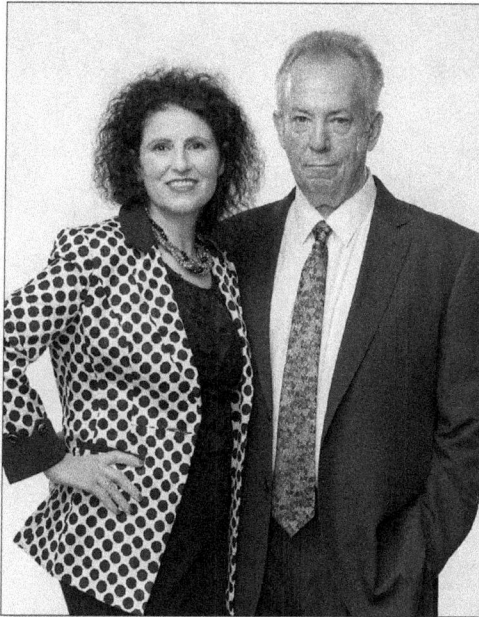